THE
HOT
TOPIC

THE HOT TOPIC

A life-changing look at the Change of Life

CHRISTA D'SOUZA

CB

First published in 2016 by
Short Books, Unit 316, ScreenWorks,
22 Highbury Grove, London, N15 2ER

10 9 8 7 6 5 4 3 2

A CIP catalogue record for this book
is available from the British Library.

ISBN 978-1-78072-267-2

Printed and bound by CPI Group
(UK) Ltd, Croydon, CR0 4YY

Cover design: Two Associates

Cover photographs: Jenny Lewis

To Nick, Flynn and Django.
And my mother for having me.

CONTENTS

INTRODUCTION

What do human beings, killer whales and gall-forming aphids* have in common? The menopause. In other words, unlike almost every other recorded species (with the possible exception of pilot whales), we all go on living well after we stop being able to have babies. From an evolutionary perspective, this has always been a conundrum. What *is* the point of living if not to reproduce one's genes? And yet here we have it: us, killer whales and gall-forming aphids* doing precisely that.

---

* Scientific name: *Pemphigus* spyrothecae. Small soft-bodied insects that produce abnormal growths similar to benign tumours or warts on the plants on which they live and feed.

Female killer whales, who stop reproducing at about 35 yet live till around 90, are far from redundant, not just teaching the grandkids how to hunt salmon but being total stick-around Italian mamas to their sons throughout their adult lives (apparently there is a 14-fold increase in the death rate of male killer whales if their mothers die).

Let's look too at the vital role the menopausal gall aphid plays within the colony. As a female loses its ability to reproduce, it starts transforming itself into a kind of suicidal glue-bomb. Once the transformation is complete it goes and sits outside the gall, or hive, and protects the rest of the colony by glomming itself onto potential predators.

Funny this. I have a mischievous writer friend called A.A. Gill, who quipped, when he heard I was embarking on a book about menopause, 'So the first two-thirds will be brilliant, the last not so much?'

Yes, well. Go look at the aphids. Which may (bar the suicidal bit) be the underlying message of this book. Because one of the best things about writing it was discovering the cold, hard scientific evidence that, from a brutally reductive evolutionary perspective, there *is* a reason for us being around. God, if you believe in him, did have a purpose for us other than looking pretty and reproducing; all those self-help gurus banging on about finding one's inner goddess and reigniting the fire within *did* have a point, while Japanese and Mediterranean societies that revere older women could teach us *more* than a trick or two.

Another thing. Did you know that the word 'climacteric' (what the Victorians called it), aside from meaning 'critical stage' also refers to the process of fruit ripening after it has fallen off a tree? A no-brainer, really. Wouldn't anyone prefer the juicy just-about-to-turn fig on the ground to the hard green one you have to yank off with both hands?

And yet. Those of you who are as old as me (55½) will remember the patronising Virginia Slims ad campaign slogan in the 70s, 'You've come a long way, baby'. Well, we have… in a way. There's so much which used to be taboo and just isn't any more.

Sex, How Much One Makes, Religion, Who You Vote For, Hair Removal, even – these are all perfectly acceptable topics to discuss alongside the chaps at the dinner table. But *The Menopause?* I want to say it is the conversational equivalent of passing wind but do I really mean that? Perhaps what I mean is that the subject is not so much taboo as plain dull, a much worse sin, in so many ways. A little like the drab, Patrick Hamilton-esque pocket of London off the M4 where I have lived for the past 18 years, the menopause is never, I fear, going to be fashionable or to 'come up'. (Come to think of it, if the menopause were a borough, it would make a very good Baron's Court.)

The seeds of this little book were planted when the editor of the *Saturday Times* magazine, Nicola Jeal, approached me to write a piece about my own experience with it. I baulked at first. Never mind if men would read it. Would *women* read it? Moreover, do you think the average Syrian refugee mourns her reproductive years? Get over it already, and all.

But I wrote it anyway, and I'm so glad I did. The feedback, after it came out (and not just from women either) was huge and heartfelt.

Quite clearly, there were plenty of super

-intelligent, super-switched-on, super-strong women out there in their late forties and early fifties who felt similarly bereft; women who, though they knew, intellectually, that just because they hit the menopause it didn't mean they were going to be circling the drain or on their way to becoming 'roadkill' (as one New York City hormone doctor I spoke to for the piece help-fully put it), but none-theless found themselves suddenly wondering who the hell they were now and what was the bloody point? Women who, like me, couldn't remember the last time they'd been whistled at by a builder or been made a proper pass at, and found the phys-ical, somatic reality of whatever that 'thing' we once had not being available again, never being available again, surprisingly devastating. I can say this only in hindsight: it is all too easy not to

A little like the drab, Patrick Hamilton-esque pocket of London off the M4 where I have lived for the past 18 years, the menopause is never, I fear, going to be fashionable or to 'come up'.

link societal value with one's sexuality… until it is irrevocably snatched away.

There was one criticism. My friend Rosa, a West Country-based film-maker gently enquired why I hadn't said anything about male menopause. And she was right – maybe I should have mentioned it for we are not the only ones who go through a hormonal crisis at this age. Imagine the hellish ignominy of moobs? But here's the thing. *Men can still technically reproduce.* If you are looking for a section on andropause, therefore, it won't be in here. (Although I will broach the subject of infertility and menopause. If you can't have, or indeed never wanted, babies anyway, does menopause matter less? Maybe it matters more.)

Somehow the point when you stop getting your period is as symbolically huge as when you first get blood in your knickers. It is very much not, as I thought it might be, a mere existential *crise*. The hot flushes, the racking insomnia, the torturous restless leg syndrome (all of which, for me, hit like a brick, within the space of barely a month) are the irreversible concrete manifestations of a chapter finishing where it had once begun. And, however much you think it won't matter, believe me, it will.

But it is not all bad. For one thing, we are not what you'd call a minority. Menopause affects half the population and, as I write this, more than a third of Western women are going through it. After the year 2030, they estimate that there will be a whopping 1.2 billion of us who have gone, or are going, through it (which is 10 per cent of the global population); and that 25 million women will go through it the year after that.

At the beginning of the last century, the average life expectancy for a woman in the UK was 48.5 years. According to the latest figures published by the National Office of Statistics, the average life expectancy for women by 2030 will be 90. If you are reasonably well off and in good health, the number, obviously, will rise. That means, if I live to 100, and there is no reason, statistically, why I should not (according to Professor Rudi Westendorp of the University of Copenhagen, the first 135-year-old has already been born), I'll have spent nearly half of it being post-menopausal.* If that is not a reason to think of it as the *next* rather than the *final* stage, what is?

Meanwhile, as women live longer, the relative time we spend being reproductive gets shorter and shorter. Might it be possible to see that febrile, fertile era between the ages of around 12 and 50 as a kind of blip? Might the time when we are at our most authentic (or as Simone de Beauvoir put it, the time when we most coincide with ourselves) be when we are either girls or old women – that is, are we at our true peaks when our fertility isn't messing with our heads?

For a second thing, why suffer if you don't need to? Just like you can have a nice sedative for a colonoscopy or an epidural before having a baby or a tooth frozen before it is drilled, so too are there ways, hormonal or otherwise, to take the edge off. You're not going to get a medal after all, however stoically you approach it.

Listen. Maybe you want to be butch about it and handle that edge and hopefully come out the

---

* The goalposts for menopause have not changed. If you were born in the 17th century and survived childbirth, you could expect to stop ovulating in your late forties, too.

other end stronger and wiser, which is perfectly fine too. Look, I laud women who, for whatever reason, get through the Change without hormones. I thought about coming off them myself for a month in a human-guinea-pig sort of a way because it seemed unfair, while writing this book, if I didn't. See chapter 6 for why that just wouldn't have worked for me.

Maybe we need to reclaim menopause, rebrand it in a more positive light and look forward to feeling the feeling as opposed to praying we'll just 'sleep' our way through it, as quite a few women proudly told me they did. Indeed, there is a school of thought, which I'll explore later, that claims having hot flushes is actually good for the brain, furthermore that they may have a positive 'halo' effect on the people around us.

As Germaine Greer pointed out in her fabulous if long-winded 1991 treatise *The Change*, 'The goal of life is not to feel nothing. The climacteric is a time of stock-taking, of spiritual as well as physical change and it would be a pity to be unconscious of it.'

I suppose what I am throwing out here, is

the idea of choice. Choice with maybe a sense of anticipation rather than dread, though it be a very different type of anticipation from the kind you felt during the Last Change, i.e. adolescence.

So here it is. The book. What it was like for me, what it will be like for you, and other things besides. I'll meet a bunch of menopausal nuns in San Francisco; I'll go hunter-gathering with the Hadza tribe in western Tanzania and I'll sit around kitchen tables with a bottle or two of Whispering Angel and a bunch of fabulous, glamorous, over-achieving women, who have just gone through the menopause and see how *they* have dealt.

Lots of books have been written about the menopause (5741 on Amazon at last count), but if you are like me you still have quite a few niggling questions. How long does it really last? Are hormones safe if you have had breast cancer? If they are, can we take them for ever? Will they make us fat? The list goes on. Is the only thing for a menopot a tummy lift? Back fat, lipo? Should I take up a hobby? Is there a cut-off point for plaits?

Oh, Lord, and then there is the old sex thing. What do we do about that? Is it our God-given right to feel horny until we die? Or is it time to finally admit that there are those of us out there who have barely done it with our other halves for literally *years*? And that we are fine?

1

HOW IT WAS FOR ME

I say all the symptoms hit me like a ton of bricks.
In retrospect – goodness, is hindsight important
when understanding the menopause – I started
having symptoms five, six, maybe even seven years
earlier. The night sweats, for example. Now, if
you are, like me, the sweaty type (my children are
hugely sweaty, while my other half barely sweats
at all), it's not something to panic about, waking
up with prune-y finger pads and a sopping
nightie. So I didn't pay much attention. Neither
to having to pee up to six times a night. Because
that's a psychological thing, right? You think

about it and you have to go – it's the Investment Wee syndrome to the power of, well, six.

Plus my body had begun to feel different. Not bigger, exactly, more like I had added some extra duvet 'togs' to it. For the first time ever, I noticed, I had *back fat*, with pouches of flesh sprouting around the sides of my bra strap. Meanwhile, when I looked down at myself in the shower all trace of hip bone had disappeared.

But then, perhaps, in my old age, I just was eating more food and drinking more alcohol. And, back in the olden days, where the latter had always been helpful in cancelling out the former, now it did to me what it did to everybody else: it made me pig-out.

Regular blood tests, which I'd been having ever since getting clear of breast cancer in 2008, confirmed the inevitable. My levels of oestrogen, progesterone and follicle-stimulating hormone (FSH), the troika of female hormones that regulate our reproductive cycles, had been steadily descending. On the other hand, it's remarkable how dim one can play to oneself if one desires. It was obviously just my body pushing the 'fuck it' button after years of being such a career dieter/ drunkorexic. Maybe my gut had started to revolt against all the red wine that had been sluiced into it before it got any solids. Maybe my zaftig genes had finally decided to show my brain who was boss. That's all it was.

And anyway, didn't two litres of water a day and a mild obsession with hot yoga mean something? Might I belong to a new generation of women who were too fit to get the menopause? The ideation that I was a rare medical anomaly had particular traction, I found, at this point of my life.

Besides, I was still getting my period. Way beyond other people my age. Oh, *boy*, was I still getting it. Getting technical here, after I hit 50, they became not only regular and closer together but almost Roman candle-like in their heaviness, a gynaecological indicator, as it turns out, that everything is gearing up for that one last chance to sprog before it is too late. Sometimes my other half would catch me stripping the bed yet again and roll his eyes. Which made me feel guilty on the one hand and cross on the other. It reminded me of a famous article Gloria Steinem wrote in the October 1978 issue of *Ms* magazine called 'If men could menstruate'. In it she imagined how it would become an important ritual for the beginning of manhood accompanied by lavish celebratory dinners and presents; that there would be a National Insitute of Dysmenorrhoea; medical funds for heart disease would be diverted into research into cramps; and lesbians would be told all they needed was 'a good menstruating man'. Brilliant. If *only* you guys knew what it was like.

And then, whooomph, they stopped. Just like that. The summer before last was the last summer I got my period. From that day on, I never got another (not a natural one, anyway). No more sitting down for a wee, looking at the gusset of my knickers and being able to go: aha, that's why I've been such a cow for the past few days. My 'woman', as some phenomenally successful Hollywood stylist I once interviewed insisted on calling it, had gone for ever. And, though I should have been grateful that I had made it this far, relieved I didn't have to play the old wad-of-toilet-paper-in-an-emergency trick any more, all I could do was mourn its passing. Its absence every subsequent month and the cartons of unopened Tampax sitting there balefully on my bathroom shelf gathering dust were such concrete irrefutable proof I had passed into the 'final stage'.

It got worse. Because then came all those symptoms I ludicrously assumed I'd be spared. Hot flushes. Palpitations. Hardcore insomnia, alleviated not one tiny bit by zopiclone. The *complete* absence of desire, as if it had been snatched, like a rug from beneath my feet. You'd think, in mitigation, the hurty bosoms and the crankiness would go after you stopped menstruating. But in my case they hung around like students who never graduate or unwanted stragglers at the end of a party. Compound that with the fact that my eldest son had suddenly gone from being 5ft nothing to over 6ft and had developed this habit of picking me up every time he wanted me to stop talking... And oh, Christ, was I beginning to fully intuit the meaning of 'old' and 'helpless'.

The biggest 'surprise'? Probably hot flushes, though thankfully they mostly happened in bed, just after turning out my light. There was, however, one notable exception. A birthday party in a very swanky members' club in Mayfair, London. Italian waiters in white coats shaving truffles onto the risotto; young women in head-to-toe Chanel, that kind of thing. And suddenly, this heat, out of nowhere, rising, rising from my solar plexus to the roots of my hair, my face pulsating like a sore thumb in a Tom & Jerry cartoon. In a funny perverse sort of way, it was fascinating that my body was able to do this, without me being able to intervene in *any way*. But the mortification of having to keep dabbing at my upper lip and eventually having to get up, dripping, in my sleeveless summery dress and go outside, cancelled the wonder of it big time.

Remember David Reuben, MD? The forward-thinking guy who wrote the 1972 No. 1 bestseller *Everything You Always Wanted to Know About Sex...But Were Afraid to Ask*? Well, this was his description of a menopausal woman: 'Not really a man, but no longer a functional woman.' But he was wrong, just like he was wrong about douching with Coca Cola being an effective contraceptive. A hot flush doesn't make you feel more like a man, or at least it didn't right then. It merely made me feel the way I had done as a new girl at school, forever in fear of getting called up in class in case I blushed: powerless and increasingly fearful of group situations...

2

WHAT IS ACTUALLY
HAPPENING TO YOU

Ignorance is bliss but knowledge is power. If you know what is happening to you, or what is going to happen to you (and being crap at biology I never really did), it might make the process less of an affront. So here goes.

Menopause – from the Greek *men* (month) and *pausis* (cessation) – was a term coined by French physician Charles Pierre Louis De Gardanne in 1821 (*la menespausie*) to mean the definitive cessation of menstruation. It is caused by a decrease in oestrogen, the female sex hormone that makes our ovaries produce eggs, although it is worth noting here that our adrenal glands, our muscles and our adipose tissue, i.e. fat, continue producing oestrogen throughout our lives. (This may be the reason why women who are overweight or super muscly often suffer less from hot flushes and osteoporosis.)

How long does the menopause last? Well, if you go by the book, just one day. Technically speaking, it occurs exactly 12 months after your last period, and can therefore only be charted retroactively, which makes it an irritating Chinese riddle from the start. In reality, the symptoms, such as hot flushes and anxiety, can last up to 30 years. (An interesting aside: in the West our most common menopausal symptom is hot flushes. In Japan it is shoulder pain. In India it is declining vision.)

Most of us start experiencing these symptoms between the ages of 45 and 55 (though Aristotle wrote of it starting at 40), with 51.4 years being the mean age of occurrence. Peri-menopause refers to the time when those symptoms start to the 12 months after your last period; post-menopause to anytime after that, but this is misleading as some women experience symptoms as many as 10 years, if not more, after they stop bleeding for good. Of course, since life expectancy was lower in previous centuries, many women didn't even make it to menopause, but it would be quite wrong to think of it as the 'luxurious' by-product of modern medicine and improved living conditions. If you survived the rigours of childbirth in the 18th century, or indeed if you remained childless, chances were you'd make it to menopause and beyond. In fact, as a condition, the Victorians were all over it like a rash, often chucking women in asylums who exhibited symptoms.

As well as causing our ovaries to produce an egg each month, oestrogen protects against a whole myriad of ailments, including heart disease, osteoporosis, memory loss and even Alzheimer's. (When we have too much of it, conversely, or rather when it is not balanced with the correct amount of progesterone, the hormone that helps line the uterus and maintain pregnancy, we may be more susceptible to breast cancer, but more, much more on this later.)

Oestrogen is also responsible for regulating the hypothalamus, a corn-kernel-like section of the brain that controls, among other things, thirst, hunger, sleep, desire and body temperature. When oestrogen levels fall, a false message is sent to the hypothalamus, indicating that the body has overheated, and in response the hypothalamus tries to cool it down by rushing blood to the surface and inducing us to perspire. Hence the hot flushes and night sweats. (Sweat itself, which is secreted by the apocrine and eccrine glands, is odourless. Only when it is acted upon by bacteria and other volatile acids does it becomes whiffy and it is the substance that the apocrine glands produce that

You could almost call it a pathology, the ability I have to smell smells seemingly unsmellable to the average human nose... If I were a dog I'd almost certainly have a little coat on my back and be employed in an airport.

bacteria love to convert into something particularly noisome. Interestingly, East Asians have fewer apocrine glands than we do – the reason, perhaps, that they mostly think we Westerners stink.)

Another benefit of oestrogen is that it produces collagen which not only keeps our skin relatively wrinkle-free but stops us peeing our pants. It does this by bolstering the walls of our vaginas and urethral tracts (Yup. Doing star jumps on the trampoline just got even worse). It also keeps them slightly acidic to ward off bacterial infection. As oestrogen levels fall, the vaginal walls become thin, dry and more alkaline, not just making sex hurt and peeing a full-time career, but making us more prone to urinary tract infections… and, ipso facto, not being quite as, um, fresh as we used to be down there. Well? Correct me if I am wrong, but wouldn't an unhappy vagina and increased propensity to sweat automatically have an impact on the way you smell?

Okay. Can we just stop here a second? Because I have to declare an interest. One of the characteristics of ageing is that we are supposed to lose our olfactory acuity, males more so than us, which is why once our menfolk hit a certain age we need to tell them to cool it on the cologne front. But has that happened to you yet? It certainly hasn't happened to me. You could almost call it a pathology, the ability I have to smell smells seemingly unsmellable to the average human nose. Not out-and-out phantosmia (the medical condition which can keep sufferers housebound) but if I were a dog I'd almost certainly have a little coat on my back and be employed in an airport.

As a demographic we are still deemed too dull for any significant studies to have been conducted around this delicate subject. And scent, let's face it, is a tricky one to be objective about. But if fertility has a smell – and there is good evidence to suggest that it does, men being more attracted to us when we are ovulating and so forth – would not the sudden lack of it act as a repellent?

Might that dreaded cloak of invisibility everyone talks about have an actual odour, and might my sniffer-dog-like abilities have enabled me to detect it? I remember thinking they probably had when I used to visit someone in Wandsworth Prison back in the 90s while working on a story. It wasn't that the guy (convicted of rape, public school educated, in his early twenties, but that's another story) smelt of sweat, not at all, he was actually scrupulously clean; it was more as if he smelt inanimate, like an uncared-for piece of furniture, almost, rather than a human being.

The author Helen Simpson writes about this beautifully in her story about the menopause, 'Arizona':* 'Nothing awful,' one of the characters muses after attending a concert where the audience was mostly older women, 'just the subdued but unmistakeable smell of underwashed jumpers and hair that had been left to go an extra day. They weren't expecting anything.'

According to Tim Jacob, Professor Emeritus of Cell Physiology at the School of Bioscience at Cardiff University, the power of smell, or the lack of it, is a 'huge unexplored, unexploited area'.

'The psychophysiological links between age and smell are as yet largely untapped,' he says via email, 'but it is a specialist area which is just waiting to be looked into and jumped on by

---

*Published in her new collection *Cockfosters* (Vintage, 2015), recommended to me by a menopausal friend, and which I urge *all* of you out there to read...

commerce and industry.'

To that end he has created Kodobio Sensory Therapy, a newly launched, state-of-the-art treatment that uses smell and light to help improve mood, reduce blood pressure and lower anxiety. 'It is designed to use natural sensory stimuli to alter your psychophysiological state, resulting in a healthy, happier you, better able to cope with the pressures of life.'

Bring it on, and, while he is at it, since he works with Procter & Gamble, could he spare a thought for us lot, and come up with a scent that makes us smell the way we did in our twenties and thirties? How to nail Eau de Youth exactly? What is it that we had then and that we apparently do not have now?

'The smell of sex, that's what,' says Jacob. 'Young secretory tissue, including the skin and the vagina, has a pH (acidic) and this supports a particular bacterial population. As pH changes during menopause (less acidic) this bacterial population changes and it is these little microbes that cause the odour of both the nether regions and the rest of the body.

'Much research in the 70s was dedicated to identify "copulins" – specific molecules present in vaginal secretions that triggered mating behaviour in male primates,' he goes on. 'This search was naturally extended to humans in the mistaken assumption that, as we are related to apes and chimps, we must exhibit the same biochemistry and behaviour. This turned out not to be the case. Then Karl Grammer [Professor of Anthropology at the University of Vienna, and a pioneer in human attraction and courtship research] carried out trials looking at the effects of these "copulins" on male behaviour. His lab found that of two groups of men looking at pictures of women, those smelling ovulatory vaginal secretions rated the women more attractive than those who were given a control aroma to sniff. One up to women, then. There *was* a sexual molecule in vaginal secretions.

'Perfumers have spent much time over the centuries adding compounds to perfume which resemble sex hormones or have odours similar to sex secretions or are from animal glands that have an influential role in sexual behaviour – why is this? There has been no consensus among them about what they are doing or whether they have succeeded and therein lies the hope and the clue – it is a mystery, well, for now at least.'

In answer to my question then, no, they have not come up with the scent of youth, nor have they come up with the scent of motherhood, which is maybe more to the point.

I know I worshipped that heady maternal mixture of Calèche and cigarettes my own mum emanated – and continued to do so, a little pathetically, right up until my late teens when I left home for the States.

And then I returned to London 12 or so years later, around the time I hit my thirties and my mother hit her fifties (young mum, my mum), and suddenly, she didn't smell like her any more. Same perfume. Different smell. Kind of sickly, like it wasn't sitting right – it wasn't *bien* on her *peau*. It really was the end of an era, that. Scroll forward another two decades and I suddenly found myself smelling that peculiar sickly smell again. *On me*. Different perfume. Same smell. It was one of the ways I knew I had entered peri-menopause, and the funny thing is I smelt it on another friend recently who has been taking tamoxifen for oestrogen-positive breast cancer. Tamoxifen blocks your oestrogen receptors by acting like a key broken off in a lock, prohibiting oestrogen from connecting to its receptor and therefore, hopefully, blocking cancer growth. Could there be a link? (I should say that, now that I am on the hormones, a cocktail of oestrogen, progesterone and testosterone, more, much more of which later, my favourite scent in the world – Tiempe Passate by Antonia's Flowers with a dot of Rive Gauche, possibly supplemented by Noble Isle's Rhubarb Rhubarb handwash – smells the same as it did before.)

'When oestrogen levels drop in menopause, a false message is sent to the hypothalamus saying that the body is overheated,' offers Professor Jacob. 'In response, the hypothalamus causes an increase in sweat production in an attempt to cool the body and this changes body odour. Tamoxifen, by blocking oestrogen receptors and thereby preventing it from working, induces some of the symptoms of menopause, including hot flushes, and if you look at internet chat-sites, people on tamoxifen report changes in their body odour from no odour, to changed and unpleasant odour.'

Phew. So I'm not such a nutter. Those smells may not be so phantom. If your wee starts smelling like chicken soup, or your prohibitively expensive perfume suddenly smells like eau de cheesy feet, or worse, your otherwise anosmic partner tells you you don't smell like you any more, it may not be your (or his) imagination. Oh, and another thing. Decreasing oestrogen has also been linked to a rise in histamine, which, according to at least one blog I read, smells a little like nuts. Histamine intolerance is not a recognised medical condition, apparently, but if you've been wondering what the stuffy nose, the itchy eyes and the peanut butter wee is all about... who can say that that is not what it is? Tests, schmests... sometimes actual testimonies count for more, as some doctor some-where might have, should have, said.

3

THE EXTRA TOG FACTOR

It was the summer of 2012, two years before I hit menopause proper, when it first became apparent. Friends had invited us to a significant birthday party on a boat in Capri—with a 70s theme. Christ, I hate fancy dress, but for once I felt okay about it because I had something appropriate to wear, a floaty halter-neck maxi which had always looked sort of ridiculous in London but would have been just perfect for this. It was while having a last look at myself from behind in the hotel's wardrobe mirrors that I noticed it. Overnight, apparently, I'd grown back fat. Back fat, which draped in folds like a chubby baby's from underneath the sides of my bikini top strap (and this is someone who, for all her bodily defects, has never had spare flesh there, even in her chunky teens and twenties).

That was a turning point, that weekend in Italy. From that moment on, it felt, everything subtly but surely started changing. My pants felt somehow 'friendlier' (as we used to call it at school when they crawled up your behind). So, weirdly, did all my shoes. Though I was basically the same size, my upper body felt – what's the word, moosier? And I found myself having to unhook my bras a notch, tucking fewer things in, wearing baggier tops. Without realising it, I was beginning to dress like my mother. My waist, meanwhile, which had never been a strong point anyway, I could literally feel going by the day. Going through some old photos, I found some of me in a bathing suit five or so years before I had babies. Nora Ephron was right: with the hip-to-waist ratio I had then, I *should* have been walking around in a bikini the whole damn time. What had been the matter with me? I looked fucking great, and now, well now… it was like wearing an extra duvet tog, or as one friend described it, like those padded cooler jackets you put on a bottle of wine. It wasn't just about being bigger, though. It was about not having any say over it. My body, after years of toeing the line when I told it to, obediently shrinking when I put myself on the Paleo Diet or 5:2 or whatever, suddenly had a mind of its own, almost like when I was pregnant. This powerlessness against the forces of nature made me angry as well as sad. Why was this happening to me? It just didn't seem fair.

So there I was, feeling moosier and moosier by

Nora Ephron was right: with the hip-to-waist ratio I had then, I *should* have been walking around in a bikini the whole damn time.

the day, and oh, did it piss me off. I pity my family at all times anyway, but I really, *really* pitied them in those two years leading up to my menopause proper. In retrospect it felt like being in permanent PMS, with no let-up from the water retention and rattiness and monstrously hurty boobs, not to mention this infernal thickening waist.

Hormonally, of course, it was all happening inside. If the first part of peri-menopause is when testosterone dominates, then the second part is when oestrogen is the relative top dog, both testestosterone and progesterone levels now fast dwindling away. Oestrogen is the good guy, I know, but when it is unopposed it can do some bad things. Inhibiting the production of hormones from your thyroid gland, for example, which slows down your metabolism; making you feel like you are walking in treacle, like you have lost your memory and, yes, causing you to gain weight. Oestrogen is produced in your ovaries and your adrenal glands but also in your fat cells and because of this a vicious cycle is set up. More fat cells, more fat storage, more fat cells and so on. But if you thought a decline in oestrogen – which, joy of joys, happens next – balances everything out, you'd be wrong. Oestrogen, for all the havoc it plays, has a soothing serotonin effect on our mood – it's what helps us feel calm and full after we've eaten. So when it goes, we don't even have that anymore, and are therefore hungrier than ever before. Wait. There's more. There's evidence to suggest that a decline in oestrogen decreases our tolerance for carbohydrates and affects the way our digestive systems work.

According to Gale Malesky and Mary Kittel, authors of *The Hormone Connection*, where it used to take only two hours to digest our food, now it takes more like four, which ensures higher carbohydrate absorption and therefore more insulin production (the hormone that is so nice and helpful in allowing us to store more fat). Cutting out carbs is the obvious solution – isn't it great the way, once you cut out the bread, potatoes and rice the pounds just melt away? – except that a very high-protein low-carbohydrate diet eats into the calcium our bones produce... and we need all the calcium we can get at this time of life to protect from osteoporosis.

Also to be taken into consideration is the extra cortisol your menopausal body is producing via your adrenal glands – that's the stress hormone which, in excess, sets off binging and cravings and contributes to the fat around your middle, and essentially means you haven't got a hope in hell of maintaining your weight, let alone losing it.

So then. Hot flushes, night sweats, an increased appetite and a thickening waist. What fresh hell, to paraphrase Dorothy Parker, will be visiting next?

At this juncture I'm supposed to say don't worry, it does drop off once your body gets used to its new hormonal state. But that is not what happened to me. Certainly the HRT worked wonders on the hot flushes and the sleeplessness and the feelings of doom. But it didn't give me back the body I had lost. And why would it? The fact of the matter was that I had, in the past year or so, slightly pressed that fuck it button around food. After years and years of treating the bread basket as if it had an electric fence around it, it just didn't seem worth it any more. Meanwhile, that cunning trick of drinking alcohol instead of eating food? Now I was doing what most people did, i.e. both. Was it because I had resigned myself to being a middle-aged mother, knowing I categorically, emphatically would never be on the pull again, and that I was never going to be my former self again so I might as well indulge? Not consciously. It's only in retrospect, I realise, that in that last year of peri-menopause (when more than likely my testosterone levels had diminished to zilch) the fridge-pilfering after supper had become the norm rather than the exception; and that I had been averaging the good part of a bottle of wine every single night (we will come back to that one in chapter 9).

What felt extra demoralising was how all the exercising I was doing to mitigate, all the Tube escalators and hot yoga I was doing... wasn't having any effect at all. But then, as studies continue to prove, you can do all the hot yoga and treadmilling and soul-cycling you like, but it's not in itself going to make you lose weight. In fact, it may even increase it (the thought being that if you increase your activity, you increase your appetite and compensate by eating more food). Fit and fat. We all know that one.

'Physical activity is crucially important for improving overall health and fitness levels, but there is limited evidence to suggest that it can blunt the surge in obesity,' public health scientists

Richard S. Cooper, MD and Amy Luke of the Stritch School of Medicine at Loyola University, Chicago, wrote in the *International Journal of Epidemiology*.

'...This crucial part of the public health message is not appreciated in recommendations to be more active, walk up stairs and eat more fruits and vegetables. The prescription needs to be precise: there is only one effective way to lose weight – eat fewer calories.'

Fewer than ever. For, once we women hit our fifties, we only need around 65 per cent of the calories we needed in our twenties. This is because every year over the age of 40 our Basal Metabolic Rate (BMR) – the rate at which we burn off calories – slows down. Meaning, if we ingest 1000 calories before the menopause we will burn about 700 of them and store around 300. Post-menopause we may store 700 while, gulp, burning only around 300.

But is it all bad? It is not. Whether it is the HRT or my body settling into menopause or a combination of both (or neither), two years on I do not have the appetite of a pre-menstrual teenager any more.

A modicum of control has definitely been regained since those ravenous peri-menopausal years, now that I know exercise on its own is not going to make me thinner. Meanwhile, I find myself liking it, loving it, actually, for very different reasons. How come I never realised it was such an effective way to get me away from all the traffic in my head? Is this what they call mindfulness? Because if it is, then, finally, after ploughing mindlessly through all those mindfulness manuals… I get it. Another thing to take on board: exercise increases muscle mass and muscle takes more calories to burn than fat. But you knew that.

It is true I cannot fit into the clothes I fitted into at my thinnest pre-menopause and I feel a little weird these days in skinny jeans if my bottom isn't covered. But then maybe skinny jeans aren't appropriate for a woman who is four years shy of 60 anyway?

Believe me, the menopause is a great time to re-evaluate your wardrobe, to throw out those things you've let languish there in the vain hope that once you lose that pesky spare tyre you'll be able to wear them again. Time to re-evaluate the

10-day juice fasts and the spenny detox retreats as well. If you have been to one you will know the uniquely joyless experience of drinking your 200th cup of herbal tea in some fancy-schmancy hotel room while staring miserably out at some Toblerone landscape, willing the week to be over. All for what? Maybe two kilos? Which we will put on, and then some, within a fortnight? And sisters, the time wasted on self. At this stage of our lives, when we haven't really got that much left to make the world a better place than when we entered it, I mean, it seems almost unholy.

Not that you need to give up on yourself. Not at all. Those ladies in that poem 'When I Am an Old Woman I Shall Wear Purple' who 'grow more fat... and eat three pounds of sausages at a go' – they are not us. (Which reminds me. I must stop wearing my prescription sunglasses in the cinema. There is a difference between eccentric and mad. As P. J. O'Rourke once said: 'Never wear anything that panics the cat.')

There is a difference, too, between taking pleasure from eating, full stop, and taking pleasure from eating because it feels like there is nothing else to take pleasure from any more. If, like me, you've always been a Labrador on the food front as opposed to a cat, if it is your natural inclination, if no one is looking, to plate-lick, then, to be brutal, it is probably time to get a grip. Overeating, especially on the baked goods front, isn't just bad for us physically, it may also make us sad. According to a study by the Department of Psychiatry at Columbia University, a diet high in refined carbohydrates with very high glycaemic indices (e.g. white rice, white bread, processed cereals and soft drinks) might lead to a greater risk for new-onset depression in post-menopausal women.* Other studies show that obesity in the menopause may be linked to heart disease and breast cancer. Being fat isn't good at any stage of life for anyone. But it is particularly injurious for us women in menopause.

I am sad, however, when I think of how much time I have spent as an adult in 'if only' mode, wanting to mould myself to clothes as opposed to the other way round, fantasising about and

* *American Journal of Clinical Nutrition*, Aug 2015.

sometimes even splurging on clothes that will never suit my particular body shape whatever size I am. Only very recently have I come to understand that, if you pay that much money for something, it has to work for you rather than you for it.

What we must obsess about now, if that is the word, what we must take time (and money) over, is making life less, not more, complicated on the clothes front, creating a kind of uniform for ourselves, a mixture of things we have come to know via trial and error will always work for us on fat, thin, bad- and good-hair days, no matter what. It's a lovely feeling, being sartorially true to oneself. I now know, for example, what I can never have enough of – silk cashmere cardigans, cotton gauze check shirts, midi-length A-line skirts with pockets; and what there is no point in even trying on – day shoes with heels any higher than 2in. I now know, too, there is no point in buying the item that will work brilliantly when it's got different buttons / is a smidgeon looser / is dyed a different colour. Unless you've got a live-in seamstress, or are a clothes manufacturer, conditional purchases never work.

Am I there yet myself? In this serene, self-accepting super-sorted-out space? Do I practise what I preach? Not quite. It is probably time for me to get a grown-up haircut, for example. But I cannot quite make the leap yet. The jeans I can no longer fit into, I know I need to make a ceremonial funeral pyre for them (or better, give them away), but have not yet got round to that either. I am, though, looking forward – kind of – to being in my sixth decade, to getting out of my neither-here-nor-there fifties, to comporting myself as an older, elegant and not completely asexual lady. I have a few role models, too. Carine Roitfeld, 61, the former editor-in-chief of French *Vogue*. Jane Fonda, obviously. Diane Keaton – now there's someone who has perfected her look over the years. Then there is my super-trim, super-stylish friend Charlotte, 68, mother of four, author, hotel proprietor and general all-round blueprint for the sexy, cool, older English lady. She exemplifies for me that Japanese concept of Shibui. I learnt about the term from that same wonderful story by Helen Simpson, in which two menopausal women discuss whether there is beauty in ageing.

Liz likens it to flowers past their prime. 'I leave anemones in their vase for as long as I can, tulips too, for those wild swoops they do on their way out, the way their stems curve and lunge and shed soot-dusted petals. In fact I like them best at that stage.' Me too. But I think Shibui can mean all sorts of things.

My understanding of Shibui is innate, old-school cool that has been honed and polished to subtle perfection over the years. The opposite of flash or 'common', as my grandmother would have called it. Because Charlotte looks so swell (in the American sense of the word), it is comforting to hear her describe her journey through the menopause in the mid-90s while living as a single mother in a remote part of Spain, as 'at least seven years of pretty good emotional hell...

'Because I had no friends or magazines or a mother or a sister out there, I just didn't know what the hell was going on and just bashed on alone, waking up in soaking sheets and feeling all wrong. My doctor gave me antidepressants and Valium which helped a little. I'm pretty sure I overate, overdrank and smoked those few years to offset the depression, which, thinking back, I'm sure had something to do with not being fertile or feeling fanciable any more.

'But I did recover. My energy returned, so did my good spirits and it was wonderful not having monthly troubles any more. Of course now I am nearly 70 what I worry about is losing my mind not my looks.'

4

SILICON VALLEY, NUNS AND HOT FLASHES

Haight Ashbury, San Francisco's former hippy enclave with its tatty head shops and psychedelic signage and strip joints, seems an unlikely place for a cloistered convent. Yet here I am, sitting in one, waiting to meet some of its inhabitants. I am accompanying Doctor Sohila Zadran, a biotech entrepreneur whom I first heard about via my hot-yoga buddy, Ingrid.

Ingrid, who, in real life manages other people's multi-million-dollar portfolio funds, had heard Zadran speak at the prestigious Milken Conference in LA about her start-up, Igantia

Therapeutics, her pioneering research into the
menopause and hot flashes (as they call them in
the States) and had a hunch we'd get on. Here we
are then, the pair of us, me a slightly jet-lagged
55-year-old, she a beautiful 29-year-old neuro-
scientist, about to meet a bunch of menopausal
nuns.

A janitor leads us through the Lysol-scented
vestibule with its bank of gloopy religious paint-
ings (all done by the nuns themselves, apparently)
into the waiting room. The Sisters of Perpetual
Adoration is a hardcore contemplative order,
founded by nuns fleeing the Mexican Revolution
in 1928. There used to be 50 of them, now there
are only 11. Because they are cloistered – meaning
they never leave the premises except, say, when
they have to go to hospital, or buy new shoes or
the Pope is in town – there is a dividing metal
grille in the waiting room which makes it feel a
little like we are in prison.

After about 15 minutes, a door on the other
side of it clicks and in file four slightly giggly,
slightly curious nuns, all of them in black veils
and starched white habits, and, despite the hot

weather, hands tucked into their bright-red tabards as if to keep warm. There is Sister Maria (46), Sister Betty (51), Sister Carmen (54) and Mother Superior Rosa (58). Three of them are still having hot flushes – including the Mother Superior, even though she has recently undergone a hysterectomy. Sister Maria, the relative new girl, having arrived only a quarter of a century ago, is just starting her transition and therefore has not had any yet.

'But she will,' giggles Sister Betty, adding, 'and we will hear about it because we know every move- ment of each other!' – which causes more slightly hysterical giggling. While Mother Superior Rosa is of course the one in charge, Sister Betty is obvi- ously The Popular Girl, a bit of a class clown, if you will. It is hard not to warm to her immediately.

A kind of hybrid Selena Gomez and the actress Anna Faris, with the gait and build of a runway model, Zadran is not quite what I'd expected, but then we are in California. She told me, as we waited, how it took some finagling, getting these visits to happen. Endless letters to the Mother Superior, endless meetings with the Chaplain, plus a crash course in the Bible. 'I figured, as a Muslim trained in the principle of Darwinian evolution, I had one chance, which was to out-Bible them.'

But it wasn't the Bible, in the end, that got them to talk. 'Once I got the Mother Superior to start talking about her hysterectomy, they all started talking,' Zadran explained. 'It was like we were bonding over this thing women had been enduring silently. That kind of transcended everything.'

Disappointingly, nobody is ever allowed behind the metal grille, but the sisters are happy to share the details of their day. It starts at 5.15am and, apart from eating and household tasks, revolves almost

'But why do you think God gave us hot flashes?' persists Zadran. 'Do you think God is sending us messages...?'
'Oh, he's sending us messages,' asserts the Mother Superior, 'although we may not know what they are...'

entirely around prayer, meditation and the 'adoration' of Mary Magdalene. ('Able-bodied' nuns often have to pray all night to 'keep the Lord company' while the others sleep.) Exercise is limited to volleyball (which they play in special aprons) and short goes on the running machine (which, yes, they do in their habits). A little TV is permitted as long as it is religion- or news-based. They are far from fit. Indeed, as Zadran told me beforehand, they all have BMIs in the clinically obese range. But despite the typically Mexican, hardly Blue Zone diet of tortillas, bread, cereal, animal protein, trans fats and coffee – though no alcohol – they live to a ripe old age. The last nun to die here, for example, was 101 and, going by birth and death records, she was no exception to the rule.

What is this down to – 'The Hispanic Paradox' (the fact that Latinos living in the US have a higher average life expectancy than whites or Afro-Americans)? Consistency? Having a religious belief? (That's one of those famous Blue Zone tips, anyway, along with drinking red wine and eating only till you are 80 per cent full.)

Zadran, who teaches a course in ageing at Stanford, thinks it may be something else, too. Maybe longevity is 'catching'. Female longevity in particular. Maybe the presence of menopausal women in a community or family actually extends the life of the women around her. A 'halo' effect, if you will. (Does this mean we are shortening our lives by not insisting on having our widowed mothers and mothers-in-law live with us? Gulp.)

Another thing. Supposing hot flushes themselves have a trigger effect, so that when menopausal women are in close proximity, secluded from other members of the population, they can sync rather in the way female menstrual cycles can sync at boarding schools? (A throwback from when we were on all fours and came on heat, perhaps?)

Whenever Zadran visits, she has an infra-red thermal imaging camera slung around her neck, just in case anyone has a hot flush. Has anyone had any today, she asks? Yes, pipes up Sister Betty, she had one at Vespers today, and it started, as it always does, in the back of her neck, the intense heat then going on to suffuse the rest of her upper body.

Bolstering Zadran's 'triggering' theory, hot flushes have so far proved to be more frequent when the sisters are together in chapel. This is especially problematic because it is hard to fan oneself when devoutly praying. One nun, not present, told Zadran it got so bad she had to leave chapel, remove her habit and then afterwards pray for forgiveness. Thankfully, Sister Betty hasn't had to do that yet. 'I offer it up to the Lord,' she says with a cheerful shrug, 'I pray, I sweat, I carry on.'

What might be worse for her is nighttime in her 'cell' (as their individual sleeping quarters are called). The others titter as she mimics the action of throwing her blanket off, putting it back on again, throwing it off and so forth. Emboldened, she spills a little more. There are the mood swings. The irritability. And then there's the hunger. Sister Betty is *always* hungry, especially for candy. Marshmallows, apparently, are her absolute favourite. 'But why do you think God gave us hot flashes?' persists Zadran softly. 'Do you think the heat means anything? Do you think God is sending us messages...?'

'Oh, he's sending us messages,' asserts the Mother Superior, 'although we may not know what they are...'

'And you know the way I think of it?' says Sister Betty, her face suddenly suffused with a rosy glow. 'I think of it as getting closer to God, of getting closer to eternity! Some people say, "You wanna come back and be born again?" I say, "Oh, no! I want to go to heaven, to see Jesus and the angels of the Virgin Mary! We are all going to be in such awe!"'

While we are talking it becomes evident that the reason they have their hands folded under their tabards on this hottest of days is actually to aerate themselves, flapping the bib part back and forth like a fan, Sister Betty doing it more vigorously than the others. Perhaps, Zadran wonders hopefully, infra-red camera poised, she's getting a hot flush now?

For Zadran, it is all about the hot flush and has been ever since her own mother went through the menopause. 'I remember vividly her switching on the ceiling fan in the middle of winter and her going, "Sohila, you have enough science to choke a horse, you have to figure this out,'" she says. 'Now my mother is one of the fiercest, strongest women I know, and that was when something clicked. How come nobody had studied the mechanism of action of a hot flash? Could it be employed as a diagnostic? Could understanding it help us live longer? I had to find out, and it became a kind of calling.'

The pair of us are now heading towards her house in Brentwood, a brand new five-bedroom in the Mediterranean style, which she bought for herself after selling her second company and lives in all alone. But then, apparently, the dating scene out here is appalling for women.

The daughter of Afghan refugees, Zadran wanted to be a ballet dancer when she was a little girl but ended up studying quantum theory at Berkeley, and earning a doctorate in neuroscience from USC. Igantia Therapeutics is the third bio-tech company she has founded (she founded the first when she was just 23) and it has two aims. The first is to build the very first global and digital initiative to analyse and monitor ageing in women, specifically focusing on hot flashes and menstrual cycles. She anticipates recruiting over 200,000 women across the world to track their hot flashes or their menstrual cycles and is already well under way with a user-friendly Igantia app and a hashtag: #iamfury ('*igantia*' is the Latin for 'fury' in case you didn't know).

The second is to develop a series of non-prescription therapeutics for menopausal symptoms such as hot flushes, which you can buy right off the pharmacy shelf. Indeed, she and her team have just developed a peptides-based non-hormonal non-herbal nose spray to stave off hot flushes for up to 18 hours. 'Think of it as Midol for menopause' says Zadran, 'though it's tricky because intensity is super-subjective. You can't exactly rank a hot flush by numbers of drips...'

Still. Something that whacks them on the head from daytime to cocktail, with no nasties attached – can the FDA please hurry up and approve it? And should I be getting her autograph in the interim?

Like many a Bay Area techie with a vision, she

hasn't had time to buy much furniture or stock her fridge. There's a very grand traditional dining room, which her parents gave her and has never been used, and a TV. Our voices echo against the polished wood floors. While she prepares supper for us – grilled salmon, kale chips and pomegranate juice – 'I'm afraid I've always led a pretty pious exemplary life' – we chat about Silicon Valley's obsession with immortality.

Ageing, or rather *anti*-ageing, is big, big business out here. Google, for example, has invested millions in CalicoLabs, the secretive R&D company 'whose mission is to harness advanced technology to increase our understanding of the biology that controls lifespan'. Then there is Human Longevity Inc, the $70-million company founded by billionaire biologist/entrepreneur Craig Venter, the first person to sequence the human genome, whose mission involves employing stem cell therapy to extend human lifespan well into the hundreds.

Peter Thiel, meanwhile, co-founder of PayPal and the first ever investor in Facebook, has ploughed millions into the quest for immortality. It is he who supports the SENS Research Foundation, headed by Aubrey de Grey (de Grey being that eccentric, bearded Cambridge professor who sensationally claimed that the first person to live for a 1000 years had already been born). But, as Zadran tartly points out, they are all men. And none of them, it seems, gives a rat's arse about hot flushes.

'When I went to my chair at UCSF, and I told him that I wanted to do a study on menopausal nuns, because no one else was doing it, he actually laughed. Can you imagine the horror of that? He said, "This is one of the best scientific institutes in the country, and you want to study hot flushes? Why aren't you doing MS or Parkinson's?" '

The answer is that she is absolutely hell-bent on changing the way the world views the ageing woman. Even if not by the time she herself hits the menopause. 'That's what I tell my students... just to record what you can is important, and maybe 50 years from now someone else will take up the baton.'

The research that is already out there on vasomotor symptoms, i.e. hot flushes, is scant.

What there is links them to both heart disease*
and impaired ultimate cognitive outcome.** But
Zadran thinks otherwise. Could they have the
opposite effect? That is, the more hot flushes
we have, the less likely we are a) to suffer heart
disease and b) to go gaga. Hot flushes, she believes
– how often we have them, when we have them,
how long they last, what they feel like – may be
the key to why women have better longevity than
men.

'Think of it this way,' she says. 'You've had
all these dynamic hormones in your body for 50
years, the oestrogen, progesterone, testosterone,
which are all critical for learning and memory,
and all of a sudden those hormones aren't there
any more. What we think is happening is that the
brain is having to adapt to the environment and
one of the side effects of that adaptation are these
hot flashes.

'The more it has to adapt, the more efficient
it becomes,' she goes on, 'a little like when you
go abroad – the more you engage with the locals,

* Amos Pines, University of Tel Aviv, 2011.
** http://www.ncbi.nlm.nih.gov/pmc/articles/PMC2756983/

the more you can live in that environment. It's as if the brain is being put into a country with a language it doesn't understand any more because there is no oestrogen or progesterone or testosterone; the way it relearns is to heat up the body, ergo hot flashes. Now, because the brain is the most important organ aside from the heart, other areas get skimped on, such as healthy bones and supple skin, hence vaginal dryness and osteoporosis – all in service to the brain.

'The data so far is too preliminary to validate… but what we think is happening is that there is a degree of plasticity in the ageing female brain, and for me this is a piece of a puzzle, and the puzzle is: why do women live beyond the menopausal transition when it doesn't make evolutionary sense, on a resource level, apart from anything else, that they should?'

5

WHALES AND HUNTER-GATHERERS. AND JANE FONDA

Yes. Why *do* we make sense? Why do we 'turn Catherine's corner' rather than keep on reproducing, or, like chimpanzees, simply curl up and die when we finally can't? From an evolutionary point of view it is one of the biggest unanswered questions: are we to thank modern medicine and better living conditions for living so far beyond our fertile years? Doesn't the fact that life expectancy for women in 1900 was 47 and by 2000 was nearer 80 make it all kind of obvious?

You would think, wouldn't you? Intuitively,

rationally, that's got to be the answer. But then why do female killer whales become menopausal? To get more of a handle on the phenomenon of *Orcinus orca* granny, I make a visit one rainy afternoon to the University of Exeter. This is where Dr Darren Croft runs his lab at the Centre for Research in Animal Behaviour. Last summer he and his colleague Lauren Brent went to the north Pacific Ocean, just off the coast of Vancouver Island, to study the habits of killer whales in the wild. Young-seeming and delightfully woolly, with hair he keeps tucking behind his ears, 40-year-old Croft is a behavioural ecologist whose past work has involved the social networks of sharks, dairy cows and guppies. (Female guppies, he'll have you know, evolved to swim faster than males in order to escape sexual harassment.)

Typically, female killer whales become mothers between the ages of 12 and 40. But, while males usually never make it to 50, the females often live for more than 90 years. Why? Croft and Brent wanted to know. When, thanks to us humans pilfering and polluting the seas, killer whales in the wild live in a more perilous environment, arguably, than ever before?

The answer, they believe, is *information*. Older female killer whales, with their old wives' wisdom, are the ones which lead the rest of the pod to precious salmon stocks – the pod depends on her, and that very much includes her some-what namby-pamby adult male offspring. Far from leaving home once they themselves mate, they stick next to their mummies for their entire lives (and if she dies – studies have shown – so, almost inevitably, do her adult sons). This, Croft explains, provides an insight into how the meno-pause evolved in humans – primitive societies, after all, didn't write down what they learnt; they had to pass it down from generation to generation.

Which brings us to something called the Grandmother Hypothesis, a crucial evolutionary theory to get your head around if you ever thought, once you hit the menopause, you were redundant in any way.

An aside. I don't know if you ever watched that reasonably amusing Netflix sitcom, *Grace and Frankie*, starring Jane Fonda and Lily Tomlin, about two older ladies becoming soul buddies after their husbands fall in love and decide to get married. There is this particular scene in one episode where the Lily Tomlin character is trying to get the checkout guy to pay attention to her rather than a cute young blonde so she can buy a pack of cigarettes. Well, you can imagine it. He acts like she is totally invisible and at a certain point Tomlin's buddy, the Jane Fonda character, has a proper crazy-lady melt-down on her behalf. 'Do you think it's right to ignore us because we don't look like *her*!' she screams like a banshee as Tomlin wheels her out of the store.

It is preposterous and hammy and not that funny (although *chapeau* to Jane Fonda for looking so absolutely magnificently wonderful at 78. Who is her surgeon? I think we need to know). But I defy you, if you are the same age as me, not to relate. And the reason I mention it here is that it's so easy to make that leap, to think that, because we cannot offer the world our sexuality, then ipso facto we must be 'roadkill'. And here we have some pretty cold proof that we are not.

The idea that we have biologically adapted to the menopause, or 'premature reproductive senescence', and are not living beyond our fertile years simply as a by-product of better medicine and kinder living conditions, was first posited in 1957 by the evolutionary theorist George C. Williams. His then revolutionary theory was that the menopause, far from being a sign of decrepitude, was a positive evolutionary adaptation. His argument was that by helping to forage for food while her daughter was breastfeeding, providing wisdom and caring for her grandchildren, unencumbered by pregnancies or infants of her own, the older non-fertile female, i.e. the grandmother, increased the chance of passing her genes on to the next generation.

Which is where anthropologist Kristen Hawkes, a pioneer in the study of hunter-gatherer foraging strategies, comes in. In 1985 she and her team went out to study the Hadza tribe in northern Tanzania, one of the few surviving hunter-gatherer groups left in the world besides the Ache in Uruguay and the !Kung in the Kalahari desert, and as such one of the last windows into the way we lived at the dawn of civilisation.

It was while observing the crucial role that

older women played within the tribe in collecting food and caring for their grandchildren that she co-developed something called the Grandmother Hypothesis, that is: females have evolved to live beyond their reproductive years to help care for their daughters' children and in doing so allow those daughters to wean their children earlier and therefore bear more offspring. In passing down their longevity genes to those children, human lifespan increased.

According to Hawkes, earlier weaning and longer childhood (as opposed to later weaning and shorter childhood in chimpanzees, our closest relatives) are what underlie subsequent important changes in human evolution, and these things couldn't, she argues, have been effected without the role of grandmothering.

Grandmothering, according to the hypothesis Hawkes favours, provided the context to make us more dependent on each other socially, to engage more with each other, which in turn gave rise to 'a whole array of social capacities that are then the foundation for the evolution of other distinctly human traits, including pair bonding [rather than mating with whoever when we are on heat, like chimpanzees], bigger brains, learning new skills and our tendency for cooperation.'*

'If you are a chimpanzee infant, you don't have to worry about your mother's commitment – it's your birthright to be your mother's central concern until you are weaned,' Hawkes explained to me on the phone from the University of Utah where she now holds a professorship. 'But if there are overlapping independents [that is, other children to tend to besides you], you have to make more of an effort to be noticed. Being canny and cute and solicitous and *needy* [my italics] will make a huge difference to your survival.'

This hypothesis** has since been contested, but was given a big fat boost four years ago by a mathematical computer simulation which showed that, even with the weakest addition of grand-mothering, ape-like life stories became human.

---

* http://archive.unews.utah.edu/news_releases/grandmas-made- humans -live-longer/
** Supported by Hawkes but originated by Sarah Blaffer Hrdy in her book *Mother Nature: Maternal Instincts and How They Shape the Human Species* (Ballantine Books, 2000).

Conversely, when the grandmothering input was taken out, those life stories stayed ape-like.

The implications of which are pretty huge. Could the menopause be the key to human consciousness? Without its existence might the human race not have evolved? Meanwhile, what must it have been like to be menopausal 1000 years ago? (And yes, if you made it through child-birth, there was a significant chance you would experience it). Was it better for us then, or worse? What did it feel like? And what does the role of the prehistoric woman *d'un certain age* tell us about civilisation now?

To find out, I've decided to put my camping phobia to one side and and go hang out for a few days with the Hadza myself.

Here I am, then, in Tanzania, bumping along a dirt track in the back of a Land Rover towards Mukengelko, one of the temporary Hadza settle-ments in the Yaeda Valley on the western side of Gideru Ridge. Numbering less than a thousand people, the Hadza or Hadzabe are a nomadic indigenous people, whose homelands are scattered around Lake Eyasi on the floor of the Central Rift

Valley and the Serengeti Plains. Because of safari hunting and neighbouring tribes encroaching on their lands, game sources have dwindled considerably since Hawkes et al were out here, and they have had to supplement their diet with modern foodstuffs in order to survive. But there are still around 200–300 who live and subsist in almost exactly the same way we did thousands of years ago before agriculture was invented.

About 20 minutes' drive from base, our guide Mika spots a Hadza couple he recognises, on the 15-kilometre walk from Domanga camp to Buluku. Because they are a nomadic tribe they have few material possessions and carry everything they own – bows, arrows, a few tools and maybe some berries picked earlier in the day – on their backs. It's a lesson in de-cluttering one's life, it really is. In fluent Swahili, Mika, who is the grandchild of missionaries and was brought up in the bush, offers them a ride and they both get into the back, looking with neither friendliness nor hostility at the two new white folk or 'mzungus' (myself and a photographer) in their midst.

Right from the get-go it is clear that Tausi, the wife, who has borne her husband five children, calls the shots. She has decided they are not going to get dropped off at Bukulu but are going to come all the way to Mukengelko with us in order to get some tobacco. Enthusiastically, I proffer a couple of packs of Camels that I bought in Duty Free having been told that, above almost everything else, the Hadza absolutely adore to smoke. Her husband takes them, but not with the effusive gratitude I confess I was expecting. See, what the Hadza love even more than tobacco is weed.

I ask Mika how old Tausi is – to me she looks my age, 55, maybe a bit younger were it not for her filmy eyes – but he doesn't know and, more importantly, neither does she. With no calendars or clocks, why would she? But she guesses around 45. She's done with having children; most Hadza women give birth to their last child in their forties. Probably because they eat less than European women, the median age for starting menopause among Hadza women is around 43.4 years compared to a median age of 49.6 for European women. Having made it to her forties, Tausi can easily expect to live into her mid-sixties and will probably survive much longer.* Statistically, her husband will die before her. Our guide tells us that many of the older Hadza men, less nimble on their feet, die falling out of baobab trees while foraging for honey. Placated with a small amount of weed, which she ties into a little knot in her kanga (reminding me of Marie Antoinette hiding her diamonds in her petticoats, in a way), Tausi sternly decides for the pair of them that they do not need to go to our camp, after all, and they both get out at Bukulu.

The following morning we are up at 5.45am when the air is cool and the sun is yet to rise: it is too hot to hunt or forage in the heat of the day. Historically, the Hadza have never experienced famine and do not see the point of rearing cattle or growing corn, which may or may not yield a return, depending on the weather and

* Frank W. Marlowe, *The Hadza: Hunter Gatherers of Tanzania*. (University of California Press, 2010) & Nicholas Blurton Jones, *Demography and Evolutionary Ecology of Hadza Hunter Gatherers* (Cambridge University Press, 2016).

environment. In this sense, they are the ultimate example of living in the present, never hoarding, always believing that there will be enough to go round the following day. And in comparison to, say, the Masai, whose herdsmen in their traditional red robes we kept seeing on the road from Arusha, they seem downright modern.

Despite a deep-seated fear of insects, and a low to mid-level of panic that a hyena or honey badger would smell the protein bars at the bottom of my bag and find its way into my tent, I find I have slept well and dreamt cinematically. After drinking the delicious locally produced coffee out of plastic cups round the fire while watching dawn break, we embark on foot on the three-kilometre journey back to Bukulu, a mere leg-stretch to the average Hadza tribesperson who is used to walking 50 kilometres or more a day.

When we arrive, a group of women, including Tausi and Elena, a young-looking girl who is suckling a child, are sitting outside a hut shaped like an upside-down nest, constructed of twigs and long grass, its gaping holes plugged up with bits of cardboard and material. These are the temporary shelters the Hadza, with their exemplary invisible footprints, are known for, melting away to nothing when they move on. Despite the encroaching heat of the day, a fire has been lit and on its burning embers is a small bowl of murky-looking water, which Elena collected from our camp last night.

Aside from Tausi and Elena, there is Hadiya, a smiley, pretty woman married to Yasaneda (Hadza for 'pothead', hah). Then there is Herta, Elena's mother, to whom the baby verging on toddler is constantly passed back and forth, the moment it struggles or utters the slightest whimper. Herta has three grandchildren in total and good-naturedly likens them to sacks of corn. Once they are partially weaned, she says, on her back they go. At no point does the toddler have reason to cry. How different to the lot of a Western baby who is left alone in his or her cot for hours courtesy of Gina Ford-style scheduled feeding, or plonked in a nursery before he or she can talk. There's a link here, as to why there is no word for 'depression' in the Hadza language, I'm sure of it. In many ways, being the child of a hunter-gatherer, or indeed any primitive society where children are treated a bit like backpacks, must be one of the most secure, confidence-building experiences in the world.

Like the couple yesterday, the women are not that fazed by our appearance on the scene. They are used to anthropologists studying their ways and the growing hordes of galumphing ethno-tourists and *National Geographic* crews wanting to take their pictures.

The men, meanwhile, are gathered a couple of feet away and are doing what they do best, shooting the breeze while melting their spear-heads in the fire to resharpen the tips; inhaling on their handmade stone pipes and cough cough coughing away as they take in the last remains of someone's stash.

In many ways, the Hadza aren't so unique. Chores are separated by sex. Men do the hunting, women do the gathering (the only animal Hadza women, by tradition, are allowed to hunt is the leopard tortoise). Women bitch, men boast, and when they're bored of their wives they leave them for younger models.

Meanwhile, given the increasing unpredictability

of game as a food source and the reliability of boring old tubers, it is the women's work that in the end counts. 'Twas ever thus, sigh. Really it should be gatherer-hunter, not the other way round.

On the other hand, there is something uniquely egalitarian, uniquely socialist, actually, about the Hadza lifestyle. Everything, but *everything*, from weed to meat to baobab fruit must be shared (I offer, as a gift, some beads and necklaces I brought from home, and notice, the next day, some of them on the necks and wrists of members from other camps I'd not yet been to).

The overall vibe, meanwhile, is unusually non-sexist – when Hadza women marry into other ethnic groups, they often return because they dislike the way non-Hadza men treat them. Arranged marriages are not at all the norm and young girls are encouraged to 'shop around' before committing. If a husband strays too long in another camp, he is quite likely to come back and find that his wife has taken up with someone else. Another thing that becomes evident the longer I'm with them is that no young mother is expected to go it alone; and no infant, it seems, doesn't have a grandmother around.

As we all prepare for the daily tuber-foraging expedition, Herta takes the baby from her daughter and straps it onto her back with a kanga. In single file we head into the bush, Tausi at the front, me at at the rear. On the way berries are picked and stored in kangas or eaten on the lam (my favourite are the green kongorobi from the *Grewia* bush, tangy but also oddly creamy, a little like condensed milk). Crucial to foraging for tubers, starchy yam-like vegetables that are one of the staples of the Hadza diet, is a *ts'apale*, a special pointy-ended digging stick which each woman makes for herself and which is initially used to tap the ground. A specific sound is produced, apparently, when there are tubers underneath the surface, and the older you are, the better you get at recognising it. Eureka! We come across a shady *Commiphora africana* tree with an *ekwa* (tuber)

In many ways, the Hadza aren't so unique. Chores are separated by sex: men do the hunting, women do the gathering.

vine winding up it. Time to get digging, and goodness, is it harder and less fun than it might look, having to constantly shovel the earth away from the hole and pulling with all your might to separate the recalcitrant stem from its source, sometimes buried two feet underground.

From an evolutionary point of view, the fact that tubers are a bugger to forage, unlike fruit and berries, is important. Though a crucial fall-back source of food, and far more nutrient-dense than fruit and berries, tubers can *only* be foraged by adults (little kids try; they're just not very good at it until they get bigger). So when the environment started changing all those millions of years ago, and the fruit and berry-rich forests started receding and giving way to bare grasslands, mothers with newly weaned infants had two choices. They could either stay in the diminishing forests where their infants could pick berries and fruits on their own, or go pick tubers and keep feeding their kids, which limited their chances of producing more kids and therefore adding to the gene pool. This is where females who'd stopped reproducing could prove their usefulness, according to Professor Hawkes and her team. They could forage for the tricky tubers in the increasingly dry, hostile environment, allowing their fertile daughters to wean their children earlier and therefore produce more offspring. Those who weaned their children late, taking their offspring with them while foraging, forcing them to become adult the moment they were off the breast, stayed ape-like. The ones who weaned their children early and 'exploited' the elder females' help – well, they evolved into human beings.

Amply supporting Hawkes' hypothesis is Herta, whose collection of tubers is far larger than anyone else's, including that of her daughter Elena, who is hampered by her toddler's steely determination to take her digging stick away.

But it feels as if it's not Elena's responsibility to forage anyway, as long as she's breastfeeding. Being a young mother, in an extended family situation like this, feels a lot less pressured, a lot cosier and more supported, than being a young mother in a modern nuclear one. And it is grannies like Herta who make it all work. (As Cambridge anthropologist Frank Marlowe noted, older women bring in more daily calories than any other age-sex category) .

Oh, but I bow to all of them, what with the insistent sweat bees buzzing in our eyes and nostrils and, actually, any orifice they can find. I notice Hadiya has bits of leaf stuck in her ears to keep them out, and I think, what a good idea, if I come out again, to bring some beekeeper helmets with me. We don't wait for the men. The tubers are roasted on a fire, lit in about 30 seconds by swiveling a chiselled stick or 'fire drill' into a piece of wood with a hole in it until embers are produced, and are immediately consumed. How to describe: like a very large fibrous radish, or maybe a swede, slightly sweeter when cooked, and for me (though not the Hadza) completely inedible when raw. Much tastier is the baobab fruit, which is like a cross between a coconut and unripe pear and can be pounded to make porridge and flour.

On the last day we head for Sengele, the next camp over. It is much bigger than both Mukengelko and Bukulu, with little children and mothers carrying babies randomly sprouting up out of the long grass as our Land Rover pulls up into a clearing. The menfolk are in a clump under a tree, doing some serious chilling after going out on a dawn hunt. Nothing caught today, but yesterday someone bagged a dik-dik and there was much dancing and singing at the feast, apparently until midnight. That's another thing – the Hadza, they love to sing and they love to party.

We have managed to procure a small amount of weed and give it to one of the young men, Mwapo, a bit of hero as he managed to bag a pregnant bush hyrax at our camp yesterday. Everyone, including the mothers and grannies and even great-grannies, demand their share as is custom, and Mwapo diligently metes it out.

Fifty or so metres behind some trees is a cluster of huts where the women and children congregate in the heat of the day. Among them is Mwapo's mother, who is known for having a lot to say about everything, but is uncharacteristically quiet today. Mika jokes with her, tries to ingratiate himself with her – it was with Mwapo that he was sent out into the bush by his father at the age of 13 and he thus treats her a bit like his Hadza mum – but she won't budge, sniffing dismissively and refusing to be placated. Apparently we have not brought enough weed to go round.

More amenable is Mbeke, the oldest female in the group and a great-grandmother. She sits on her heels, takes some weed from a knot in her kanga, rolls it into a cigarette and lights it with an ember from the fire. Although Mbeke is obviously well into her eighties, bowed and skinny with one eye missing, Mika explains that she is still very much part of the community, foraging, dancing and partying. When she dies, however, which cannot be too far off, there will be no sentimental ritual. The Hadza have a god called Haine, but they do not believe in life after death.

Then there is Maria (thanks to the missionary influence, a lot of Hadza have European-sounding names and are happy to wear European clothes), who is the 'Big Mama' of the group, according to Mika. A mother and a grandmother and some-where between 45 and 50, she has also adopted two orphans whose own mother recently died. A lot of the children in camp, she says, treat her as a mother figure, even if their own are alive. One of the orphans, Amina, keeps darting in and out of the hut, and shyly plays with Mika's dreadlocks while we are talking. Life was easier, Maria admits, when she was a young mother, because she got so much help from her parents. She says she works harder now than she has ever done before, but does not begrudge it at all. Yes, she has experienced hot flushes, and says that is how women know they cannot have babies any more, but the idea that this signals the beginning of the end, or that women should try to hold onto their youth, pretend they are younger than they are, rather stumps her. Why fear the inevitable? When you still have such an enormous role to play? When, without you, the whole system would collapse?

She's right, of course. But how does this relate to *me* – Christa, of London W14, who never left her children with either grandmother, not once? It's a double-edged sword, all this, isn't it? If it weren't for primitive grandmothering, we wouldn't *be* here – we'd be dying soon after having our last babies, just like our closest relatives, chimpanzees. On the other hand, the presence of grandmothers means that we've got to cope with living way past our prime... and with the grim spectre of the dreaded younger model. (To spell it out, the existence of menopausal women, i.e. grandmothers, makes younger, fertile women scarcer and therefore more prized. In that mathematical simulation I mentioned earlier, the ratio of fertile males to fertile females when grandmothering was added in jumped from 77 males to 156 males per 100 females in 30,000 to 300,000 computer years.)

Interestingly, it's the other way round for chimps; males prefer older models – well, doesn't experience count for something?

'And this is the really important question if you can tackle it,' laughs Hawkes, herself the picture of elegance at-any-age with her pixie-ish silver crop and Carly Simon-like features. 'You see someone like Gloria Steinem who's been such a tireless worker for women's rights – yet there she is in the *New Yorker* magazine in this beautiful sexy posture and you think, is *that* what women are supposed to look like at 80?

'Do I think she is a traitor? Well, in a cultural context, yes! We all know that looks matter, and there is this whole industry which ensures we keep feeling it matters; but shouldn't we be shifting these attitudes? What do we actually mean when we say Gloria Steinem and Jane Fonda look good for their age? We mean they look like they could still be fertile. But when you think of some of the components that make us human, the components that are consequences of this post-fertile stage and that allowed us to think and be the way we are, why shouldn't *they* be attractive too?... An attractiveness *outside of fertility* [my italics] is way more interesting to me. Now if you could set your cap at making that shift, you'd be doing a very big service indeed.'

6

THE CASE FOR AND AGAINST HORMONES

At the end of last summer, my mother, my younger sister and I went to Puglia, in southern Italy, for a week. The idea was to leave all the kids in London, take hand luggage only and sneak in some more baking by the pool before term started. As it turned out, it rained solidly for six days, inside and out, with all the slugs of Puglia, it seemed, taking shelter in our dank little trullo. Our trullo with no wifi and no TV. Just lots and lots of slugs which we kept sweeping out and which kept grimly coming back in. The

Some snaps from over the years...

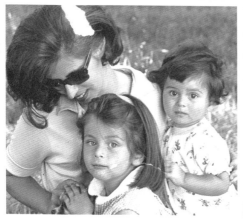

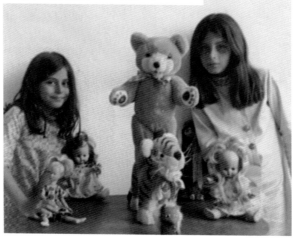

top: 1964, with my mother and sister on Hampstead Heath

bottom: 1967, my sister and I on a hotel balcony on Orchard Street, Singapore

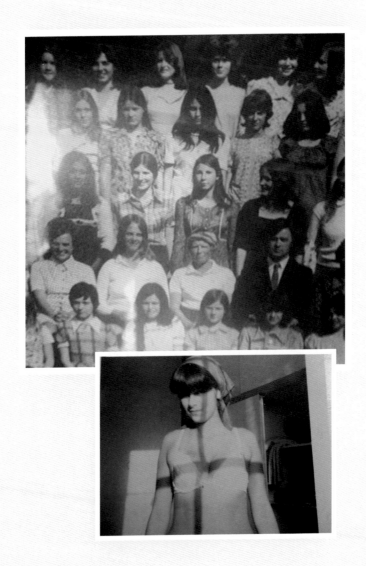

top: The 1974 Badminton School photo. I'm in the middle of second row from top

bottom: 1975, in my first wonderbra, aged 15

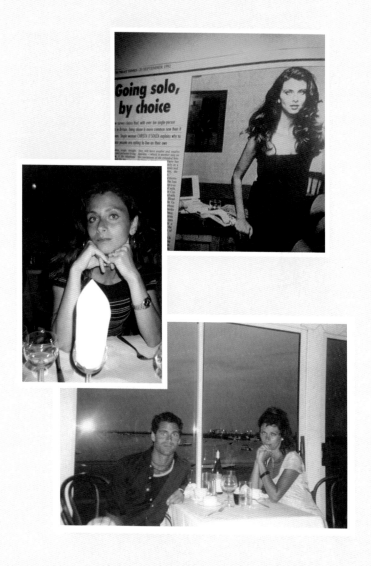

top: My first assignment for *The Sunday Times* (I wasn't actually single at the time)

middle: Ramatuelle, South of France, 1991

bottom: With my ex-husband, in Provincetown, Mass., 1994

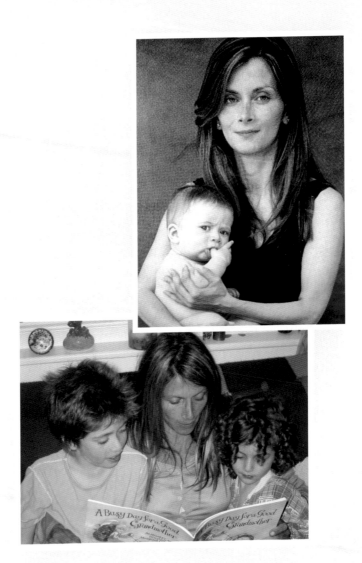

top: With my first-born, Flynn, in 1998 (he had just weed on me)

bottom: At home in London, 2005

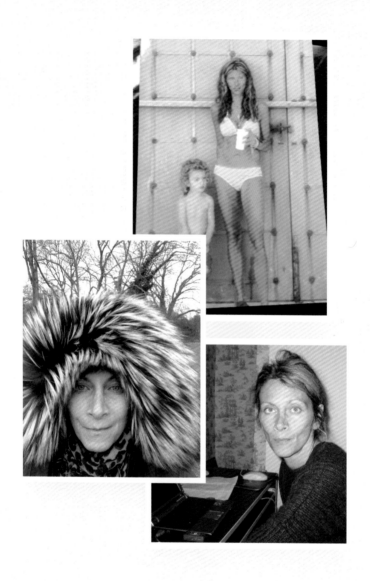

top: Mykonos, 2005, with Django

middle: 2004, in the garden at our cottage in Wiltshire

bottom: In the spare room in Wiltshire, working

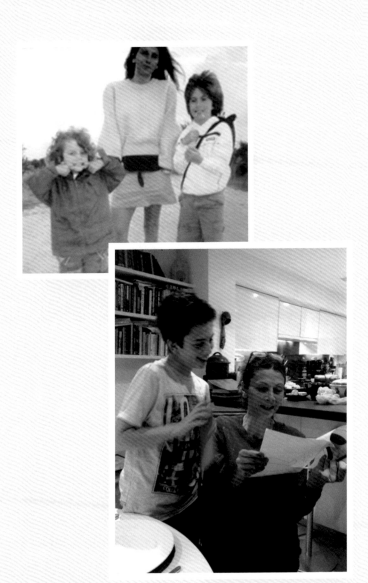

top: On White Sheet Down in Wiltshire with Flynn and Django, 2007

bottom: With Django in the kitchen, 2014

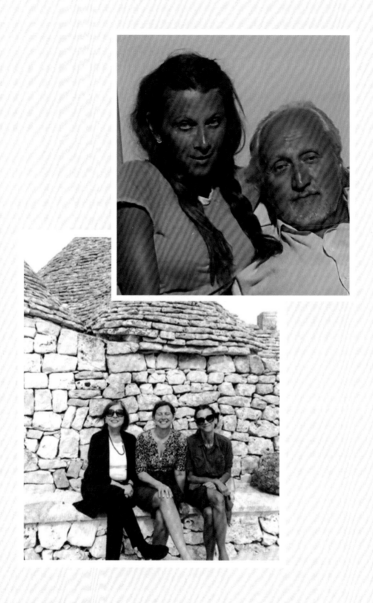

top: With Nick, partner and father of my children, summer 2015

bottom: With my mother and sister in Puglia, Italy, 2015

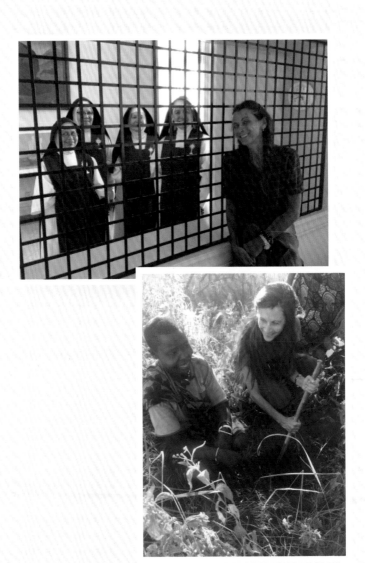

top: Silicon Valley, 2015, with the Sisters of Perpetual Adoration – menopausal all

bottom: Digging for tubers in Tanzania, February 2016

only thing to do besides reading our books (and sweeping the slugs out) was to eat and drink and talk. And goodness, did we talk. I had no idea, for example, that my mother suffered terribly during the menopause, can't even remember, in fact, when she had it (which was around the age of 53, the time she split up with her second husband). This is my mother who sailed through childbirth (always likening it, unhelpfully, to bad period pains), my mother who once lived up a treehouse in Borneo and during the 80s travelled around Afghanistan with the Mujahidin.

'Whole nights would go by where I wouldn't sleep, so I'd get up at five in the morning and just go into work. I felt this new mixture of fear and sadness, the kind where there was no bottom, no depth or safety net to it. I remember being too terrified to even let myself think about it because what if it never ever ended?'

The hot flushes, she recalled, did not last long, but they were 'intense' and debilitating. Once, she remembered, while having a walk by the sea, she became so uncomfortable she actually walked into the water with all her clothes on. Which makes her sound a little mad, I agree, but she is so... not. Adventurous, brave, unerringly optimistic, but not mad.

Looking back, she described it as a perfect storm. Our cleaning lady of 25 years left. The bolthole cottage she had been renting for years in Devon suddenly became unavailable, she was broke, more broke than ever before, being saddled with a mortgage and, yes, there was the break-up of her marriage. It was also when, after years of being 8st 4lb, no matter what, she got fat.

'I began to wonder if becoming menopausal had caused the break-up. Had I become less attractive? Is that what had happened? I went into this complete downturn for four years, wondering which was which.'

My sister Heloise, 53, another non-fusser, was similarly hit sideways when 'it' happened.

'I'd always thought, I'm *not* going to be that person who conforms to the complaining menopausal stereotype. I was the same when I was pregnant: I worked up until the night before with Polly [her first child, now 23]. My feeling was it wasn't going to affect me, because nothing affects me.' And then it happened. The debilitating hot flushes in the middle of meetings ('weirdly I didn't associate this with being menopausal, I must have been blocking it out'), the inability to sleep and, maybe most importantly, the plunge into nihilistic despair, from which she has not yet, she admitted, quite climbed out. Example. She went to the dentist recently because she had a toothache. 'He told me it was possible to save the tooth, but I just thought, what's the point? I'm old. I might as well just have it taken out. So I had it taken out.'

Quite a few of us are facing that dilemma at the dentist's: whether we are worth the hideous expense and/or bother or not. Take Orla, a 50-something account manager mother of two, who found herself unable to justify the cost of the Invisalign braces her dentist strongly recommended to mitigate the bad orthodontic work she was subjected to as a child in the 70s.

She likens herself to the 'old family Volvo, which we will keep as long as it runs well, fixing the indicators and such but don't worry about the fabric on the seats getting torn a bit and we certainly wouldn't bother with replacing the carburettor. Just no point in throwing good money after bad.'

'It's not that I want to duvet-dive or eat chocolate exactly,' my sister explained, 'but I feel if I got cancer that was inoperable, well… I've done my thing, I've lived my life. A bit like the way women thought of themselves 70 years ago, I suppose.'

Yes. Just like the eminent psychoanalyst and author Helen Deutsch who authoritatively described the menopause in her 1945 book *The Psychology of Women* as 'a partial death where everything [a woman] acquired during puberty is now lost piece by piece; with the lapse of the reproductive service, her beauty vanishes, and usually the warm vital flow of feminine emotional life as well.' Or what about iconic feminist Simone de Beauvoir and her nihilistic approach to getting older: 'Suddenly I collide again with my age…' she writes soon after her 50th birthday, in the epilogue of *Force of Circumstance*. 'That ultra-mature woman is my contemporary. I recognise that young girl's face belatedly lingering amid the weathered features. That hoary-headed gentleman, who looks like one of my great-uncles, tells me with a smile that we used to play together in the Gardens of Luxembourg.

'"You remind me of my mother," I am told by a woman of about 30 or so...'

And then, the horror at having to confront herself in the mirror. 'I understand La Castiglione, who had every mirror smashed... I loathe my appearance now: the eyebrows slipping down towards the eyes, the bags underneath, the excessive fullness of the cheeks, and that air of sadness around the mouth that wrinkles always bring. Perhaps the people I pass on the street see merely a woman in her 50s who simply looks her age, no more, no less. But when I look, I see my face as it was, attacked by the pox of time for which there is no cure.'

De Beauvoir is quoted extensively by second-wave feminist Germaine Greer, who herself, in her 1991 book *The Change,* wrote that the menopause was a time for 'mourning'. It's a great book, one of those books that should be in every school library, but boy, is there a lot of misery before you get to the chapter entitled 'Serenity and Power'.

Feminism, it seems, provides no immunity against the profound sense of loss menopause can trigger.

Back to the 21st century and my sister, though, who has always had a proclivity for 'negative fantasising'. We both have; it's a trait we inherited from our dad, but it was a shock to hear just how useless she genuinely felt. *And* how she wasn't doing anything about it. My mum, I could understand – HRT was not really part of the British vernacular back in the early 90s. But my sister, I felt, was different. What was this thing she had about suffering and bearing it when she didn't have to? They had hormones in Chard, for goodness' sake! On the other hand, perhaps she was right. Perhaps those of us on hormones are only delaying the inevitable. Isn't the only way to tackle any problem to go through it rather than around it? Maybe, dare I say it, we need to grow a pair?

A case in point is my friend Samira, 52, of Indian parentage but born and bred in the UK. 'Who knows whether my Asian genes helped me, but there will always be those women who just have to make a huge big feminine drama out of what is essentially one of the most natural things in the world,' she says. 'I'm not saying I'm not sympathetic to those who truly suffer but, if you are going to do anything in life, do it with grace and style. It's a private affair and hot flushes do not need to be announced and apologised for. And there *are* practical solutions. Can't sleep? Take Stillnacht, that's what I did, and because I knew sugar exacerbated menopausal symptoms, I cut out alcohol too. And I got through it with no problems at all. It's important that women who do have an easy menopause are not barred from saying so just in case it makes other women feel inferior. Another thing is to be a bit of a Brownie about it and prepare ahead of time. The big M can be okay, in my experience, if you don't let it sneak up on you and grab you from behind...'

'Menopause is a little like childbirth in that you know people who have been through it but you have no idea what it is really like until you are in it yourself.' So speaks graphic artist Deana, 57, ex-pat American and mother of one who, like Samira, chose not to go down the hormones route even though her symptoms were much grimmer. 'I was having hot flushes every night and they'd wake me up every damn cycle, so I'd be exhausted and cross every single morning. They came in the day as well, triggered by wine, coffee, food (yeah, pretty much everything) and any slightly stressy moment. My face would go red and it felt like I was on fire inside, but my skin would be cold. My libido went out the window, and I experienced what a lot of people talk about – a kind of disembodiment: I didn't feel *in* my body.

'The most upsetting thing was my brain switching off. I'll never forget one horrible moment at the butcher, when he told me he didn't have lamb mince. Oh my God, my entire world fell apart. I made it home and the moment I walked in the door, I burst into tears. My husband and son thought something horrific had happened to me – well, yes, it had! But I remember the look on their faces when I told them why I had been crying. Men do not understand, I guess. I would say I'm a fairly calm person, I try to take a breath before reacting and I try to go with the flow, but this little episode was *so* unlike me – I've certainly never sobbed like that at something so trivial. I felt utterly thrown off my mark – I couldn't work out a new plan for our dinner party, I couldn't stop crying, I felt helpless and I simply wanted to give up, crawl into bed and keep crying.'

She explains why, despite this very dark period, she steadfastly resisted taking hormones.

'I'm not one who rushes to pills anyway. It is like when I gave birth to my son Louis. I did it without pain relief – not by choice; I was one of the .001 per cent of women for whom an epidural doesn't take – but it was so amazing to have felt everything about it.

'Plus, I worried about what would happen once I came off the HRT. Didn't the symptoms simply return? A lot of my friends had gone on it, but I just kept thinking, I'll tough it out. If it gets too bad, I can try them. I felt that whatever I was going through was completely natural for my body and that it was important that the entire process be allowed, not suppressed.

'Of course, I had no idea that it would be another six years before the fog lifted. But I absolutely felt I did the right thing for me. I went through it fully aware of my body's changes and I can tell you, I knew when my menopause was over – I literally woke up one day and felt like my old self. No kidding. I felt centred and calm and – bloody hell, what was that? – happy!'

The idea of taking hormones? To be honest, I didn't consider it either at first. But there were a few reasons for this. The first was that in September 2007 I was diagnosed with breast cancer after finding a lump the size of a grape pip in my right breast while on holiday that summer in Greece. Only grade I, treated with radiotherapy (my oncologist said I didn't need to bother with tamoxifen if I didn't want to) and a mere verruca compared to the experiences so many of my poor friends have had with the disease. But it was cancer nonetheless and oestrogen-positive to boot, meaning that I simply wasn't eligible for HRT. HRT included oestrogen and the last thing my body needed, quite obviously, was more of it. The second is that I have always had a slight fear of hormones – it's why I never took the birth control pill for any length of time. The third was the 'embarrassment' factor. There's a rumour going round west London, of a woman, newly divorced, in the throes of passion with a new lover, and telling him the oestrogen patch on her arm was actually Nicotinell.

Also, there were alternatives. There always have been. Belladonna. Opium. Rattlesnake poison. Star anise. Lead injections. All sorts of non-hormonal substances and methods have been used to treat menopausal symptoms over the years. In 1849, one William Tyler Smith recommended a course of ice water injections into the rectum and the vagina for hot flushes, followed by the application of leeches to the labia and cervix (as reported in Louise Foxcroft's wonderful book *Hot Flushes, Cold Science*: 'His colleagues were advised to count the leeches when they removed them to make sure none was lost and left there.') The still common practice of prescribing antidepressants the moment the word menopause is mentioned in the GP's surgery is surely a legacy of the Victorian response to menopausal women, which consisted of either treating them for hysteria or chucking them in an asylum.

Black cohosh (originally used by Native

Americans), *Pueraria mirifica* (extracted from a plant found in Myanmar); Relizen (whose active ingredient is harvested from Swedish flower pollen) – these are just some of the non-hormonal plant-based formulas out there which claim to relieve menopausal symptoms, many of them to be found on the shelves of Holland & Barrett. Kinesiology acupuncture and traditional Chinese medicine have been known to make a significant difference to some women. (Watch out for a new treatment from the US called Menerba which consists of 22 herbs used in Chinese medicine and is currently awaiting FDA approval). Then there is something called 'maca', a turnip-like root found on the Andean plateaus which Peruvians have been taking for centuries. As well as balancing hormones, protecting against brain damage and relieving hot flushes, maca is supposed to increase libido and aid vaginal lubrication. Does it get you high, too, you may ask? Well, it is taken by athletes to improve performance and old people to increase vigour, so there's obviously something in it.

There are wackier solutions… knicker magnets,

for example, which clip onto your pants and supposedly emit magnetic forces that soothe the nervous system and boost oestrogen and progesterone levels while they are at it, or what about cooling jewellery, as publicised by Oprah Winfrey, literally a necklace of beads filled with cooling gel that you keep in the freezer so they are nice and cold when you put them on.

The use of actual mammalian hormones to treat symptoms of the menopause may be charted back to the 1890s when a US pharmaceutical company brought out a powder called Ovariin, made by grinding up dried cows' ovaries. By 1933, the first HRT product, Emminen, was on the shelves. It contained the urine of pregnant women (the very first form of bio-identical hormone therapy, therefore). But it was very costly to manufacture and in 1941 it was replaced by the much cheaper Premarin.

Manufactured by Wyeth Pharmaceuticals, Premarin was harvested from pregnant mares' urine and by 1992 became the most widely prescribed drug in the US. 'Keep her on Premarin' as the jaunty, hugely successful campaign, aimed at both American men and women, went. And so the popularity of HRT in general kept growing. Until, that is, the findings of the now famous Women's Health Initiative (WHI) study were published in the US in 2002.

Initiated in 1991, the WHI study was intended to examine the effects of HRT on 161,000 menopausal and post-menopausal women for a period of 15 years. The point was to prove that drugs such as Premarin and Prempro (conjugated horse oestrogens plus progesterone, introduced in the 70s when it was found that unopposed oestrogen was linked to a higher incidence of uterine cancer) helped prevent heart disease in menopausal women. But the study had to be prematurely stopped when it was found that the risks of breast cancer and heart disease were far outweighing the drugs' benefits. Suddenly, from being the course of action that every menopausal woman should take, as celebrity gynaecologist Dr Robert Wilson famously advocated in his 60s bestseller *Feminine Forever*, HRT users and prescribers were made to feel they were playing Russian roulette. The year before these injurious findings were made public,

33 per cent of women over the age of 50 were taking HRT (1.7 million women in Britain and 22 million women in the US). By the following year, that percentage had more than halved, with doctors only prescribing it in extreme cases.

As critics, and there are many of them, have since pointed out, there were flaws in the study. For one, the average age of the women in the study was 63, 12 years older than the average age for menopause. (It had already been proved that administering HRT to women in their fifties protected against heart disease.) For another, they were all given the same oral dose of Prempro (0.625mg conjugated equine oestrogens and 2.5mg medroxyprogesterone acetate versus placebo, to be precise).

But there were other studies to compound the turnaround; the Million Women Study, for example, which was set up to investigate links between HRT and breast cancer and conducted in the UK between 1996 and 2001. The findings revealed that 20,000 of the 950,000 women who took part developed breast cancer. In a joint statement, Professor Valerie Beral and Professor

Richard Peto from Oxford University said: 'HRT is one of the most important causes of breast cancer in the world and women can easily change their risk by stopping.'

Again, critics pointed to flaws, including the fact that women may already have had breast cancer when they embarked on the study. The lobby to rehabilitate HRT grows. Take the study conducted in Denmark, published in the *British Medical Journal* in 2012, which suggested that there was no increased risk of heart disease from taking HRT and that it may even protect against it. A study published in the *Journal of Clinical Oncology* in 2015 led by researchers at the Institute of Cancer Research in London found that women with the commonest type of ovarian cancer could not only safely take HRT during or after treatment, but could actually survive longer by taking it.

Meanwhile, the latest guidelines from the National Institute for Health and Care Excellence (NICE), published in 2015 in the UK, sought to reassure doctors and their female patients about the safety of HRT, and highlighted the importance of educating women about its benefits as well as its risks, to make it less of the bad guy, and to give those of us who suffer debilitating symptoms, such as having to change the sheets every day and so on (and, indeed, the one in a hundred women who become menopausal before the age of 40) more options. But the debate continues to rage, and the reputation of HRT is still very much in recovery.

Not helped, it would seem, by the rising trend for bio-identicals, an alternative to HRT about which, as I discovered, much confusion reigns...

If you are a baby boomer, like me, and have a vested interest in such things, chances are you think you know the difference between bio-identical hormones and conventional HRT. The former are the modern organic ones that are made of plant sources like wild yams or soybeans, have an identical structure to the hormones our bodies produce, and are only available through private doctors. The latter consists of the hormones they've been using since the 60s, harvested out of the groins of mares who are never allowed to lie down, are reinseminated immediately after they give birth and not given enough to drink in order to make their pee more concentrated – the one-dose-fits-all chap that your harassed NHS GP prescribes just to get you off his back. Good guy, bad guy, right?

Well, kind of, but not quite.

The word bio-identical is slightly tricky. Yes, it refers to hormones that are biochemically similar to the ones the body produces. But, although they derive from wild yams or soy, they have to be chemically synthesised in a laboratory. True, the idea of having reconstituted sweet potato in one's body is a hell of a lot more appealing than having reconsitituted horse urine (well it is for me, anyway), but the idea that bio-identicals are all-natural – as you, like me, may have been led to believe – is simply not true. Remember, too, a *lot* more trials have been performed on synthetic hormones (such as Premarin) than on bio-identicals. To further confound the issue, a lot of commercially available HRT preparations, the ones your GP might prescribe, contain oestradiol 17-beta, the natural human oestrogen, or micro-nised progesterone which is the same thing as natural human progesterone.

But then, if you hear a friend raving about the bio-identicals she has been prescribed, what she probably means is that they have been compounded for her in a specific strength (in a cream or lozenge, for example, rather than a pill) – that is, titrated, by a specialist pharmacist as opposed to being dispensed in a one-size-fits-all dose. Same medicine, different strengths.

True, the idea of having reconstituted sweet potato in one's body is a hell of a lot more appealing than having reconstituted horse urine (well, it is for me, anyway), but the idea that bio-identicals are all-natural is simply not true.

Now, there are thousands of these compounding pharmacies in the US, many of which sprung up in the wake of those worrying WHI findings back in 2002. (And as US critics argue, since their production or titration is not monitored by the FDA, there is reason to believe they are actually *less* safe than synthetic HRT such as Premarin, Prempro et al. In the UK, we have just one compounding pharmacy – though of course that's bound to change.)

'If you treat the menopause as a lack of hormones then you miss the point totally.' So declares Dr Mikael Rabaeus, head of cardiology and internal medicine at the Clinique La Prairie medical spa in Montreux, Switzerland. Founded in 1931 and made famous by clients such as Marlene Dietrich, Winston Churchill and David Bowie, it is the first medical spa in Europe to boast a clinical centre entirely dedicated to the menopause. This, by the way, was the first port of call in writing this book. 'I find when I talk to my female patients,' continues Dr Rabaeus, 'most do not qualify for taking hormones; they qualify for taking care of themselves. But then lifestyle is my main concern as a cardiologist. It accounts for 80 per cent of your risk of early death. Ceasing smoking and doing physical exercise has an excellent effect on menopausal symptoms and life expectancy in general. I also belong to the school of thought which is little convinced by a treatment you have to take for an indefinite amount of time.'

'To treat menopause, it is very important to tailor the needs to the patient,' says his colleague, Dr Thierry Pache, an endocrinologist by training, who founded the menopause centre at Montreux in the late 90s. 'I felt such shame for my gynae-cologists when I discovered the average length of a gynaecological appointment was 12.5 minutes – and that included taking your clothes off and putting them back on again. Seeing a patient about menopause requires a minimum of half an hour, and that's just the talking. There was a lot of criticism when I first started,' he adds. 'The least nasty comment I got was: "Pache, what're you doing with all these old ladies?" But this had been happening all through my training in ob/gyn back in the day. When I told my former mentors that I was interested in gynaecological endocrinology and how hormones could be regulated, they just said to me, "Listen, you are here to remove uter-uses and deliver babies. Just work and shut up."'

It is a shame that Dr Pache, who speaks five languages fluently and has won several awards for his vineyard in Argentina, only practises in Montreux. He is so full of bonhomie and so lacking in the patriarchal smugness that has always permeated the world of ob/gyn. Unlike his colleague Dr Rabaeus, he thinks hormones can be 'fantastic, if you are administering the appropriate dose to the appropriate patient. I have patients who are 75, 76, who are still using HRT. We try stopping, and back come the hot flushes.' He cites publications that reveal that having two glasses of wine a day are more of a breast cancer risk than taking full-dosage conventional HRT and says he is '*still* waiting for the paper to show me that oestrogen causes cancer. Because it doesn't exist'.

But it remains his heartfelt conviction that in general, women in Western society are overloaded with hormones, and he would never treat me, a breast cancer survivor (how melodramatic that sounds!) with them. 'I have four or five patients who have suffered from oestrogen-positive cancer like you but they are having six hot flushes an hour and they have begged me to do something about it. In these exceptional cases I have contacted their oncologists and so far they are doing perfectly well, but you, with your history, I would refuse to treat with hormones.'

He recommends, instead, a formula called Climavita Forte, which contains black cohosh (also known as *Cimicifuga racemosa*) and, as I later read up, is fantastic at treating bed bug bites. 'It can be used by women even when they are being treated for positive breast cancer,' says Dr Pache, 'and if you pair it with a good acupuncturist it has been shown to help a lot with symptoms.' But no, it will not do a thing for an expanding middle. Only four hours of exercise a day and a change in diet, he says, will do that. 'I think even Audrey Hepburn had trouble in this area,' he says sympathetically, 'but then the way a woman's body changes around menopause, a lot of men, including myself, find that rather beautiful.'

And so I flew back to London with my prohibitively expensive bundle of Climavita pills, feeling, it has to be said, rather dejected. The hot flushes were still coming thick and fast, I was imprisoned in leggings mode because none of my jeans fit, and the impotence and resentment I felt as a result were becoming increasingly hard to deal with. Why did I have to bloody go and get cancer? Why couldn't I be one of those women who felt better than well after taking HRT?

Like my friend Rosa, a successful documentarist in her early fifties, who herself had a terrible time of the menopause despite being super-prepared. After what she euphemistically calls a 'treasure hunt' of doctors, she was prescribed bio-identical HRT, and within a few days of taking it – a mixture of non-synthetic progesterone, oestrogen and testosterone – went through what she described as a kind of epiphany. 'I have to say, I didn't feel better, I felt incredible, with these real proper power surges of well-being. I mean, if hormones are bad for me, it's hard to believe because it feels *soo* flipping good.'

'Whatdoyoucallit? *Cimicifuga*? Honestly, sometimes I do despair.' This is Professor John Studd, consultant gynaecologist at Chelsea and Westminster Hospital, Professor of Gynaecology at Imperial College and former chairman of the British Menopause Society. Striking slightly of Sir Lancelot Spratt (the character James Robertson Justice played in the *Carry On Doctor* films), with his quiff of silver hair and booming patriarchal tones, Professor Studd is a world expert on the links between menopause and loss of libido, and was the founder of the very first menopause centre in this country in 1969. (The first in the world was set up two years earlier at the Groote Schuur Hospital in Cape Town, South Africa, where Christiaan Barnard performed his first heart transplant.)

Studd is also an unashamed proponent of HRT, yes, even for women like me who have had breast cancer. While I tell him about my history, he gets up from his desk and pads over to a chaise longue with his shoes off, all the while peering at me from above his glasses. I have now gotten to the bit about being prescribed Prozac for depression back in 1988 and still being on it, a quarter of a century later, at double the dose (40mg) I had taken to start with. And my history of osteopenia (that is, low bone mineral density, thought to be the precursor of osteoporosis).

'With your history of depression and low bone mineral density, of *course* you must take it,' he says and, padding back to his desk, he briskly whips off a prescription for oestrogen gel, testosterone gel and progesterone in pill form, the latter being the only one he anticipates I *might*, even at this low dose, have trouble with – but necessary 'because you still have a uterus'.

Typically, he doesn't hold back on the subject of bio-identicals. 'Such bullshit. All I can say is that we in Europe have been using so-called "bio-identicals" for 20 years. It's only the Americans who were using horse piss. Now, of course, they're waking up to the fact that they've been wrong for 30 bloody years. I wouldn't touch Premarin with a barge-pole.'

My wonderful oncologist Carmel, meanwhile, rather rolls her eyes when I go in for my six-monthly check-up and sees that I have decided to go down the hormones route. I can do what I want with my own body is her general message but, if I want her opinion, she suggests I don't. Why would I want to put more oestrogen into my body, when I have oestrogen-positive cancer? she wonders. Especially when I am already at risk by being a drinker? Is it because I want to rekindle my sex life? This social pressure that we're all under to be having fantastic sex for the rest of our lives, she sighs. It's so exhausting. Isn't there life beyond sex, at some point?

Back and forth, back and forth. Part of me feels morally weak for wanting to take the edge off. Isn't it just delaying the inevitable? My symptoms are not as bad as a lot of other women's are, after all. Not just that. Do refugee mothers in Calais complain about hot flushes and expanding waistlines? Do the majority of Japanese women? As anthropologist Margaret M. Lock posited in her groundbreaking book *Encounters with Ageing* (1995), maybe it is not just the diet of soy that accounts for the lower rate of menopausal symptoms in Japanese women; maybe it is because the menopause is seen as a natural part of the ageing process as opposed to a disease involving physical and emotional decline.

Perhaps, says Susan Bewley, Professor of Complex Obstetrics at Kings College London, and a vocal critic of the latest NICE guidelines regarding hormones, it is really a problem of culture and perception more than anything else. 'If your status was raised by menopause, if you were treated as the wise woman, listened to, regarded, if people sat at your feet listening to your stories,' she told Zoe Williams in the *Guardian* in a comment piece about reversible menopause, 'and the older men still found you very sexually attractive, what would be the problem?'

Nonsense, thinks Dr Erika Schwartz, author of *Don't Let Your Doctor Kill You,* whose glamorous Fifth Avenue practice above Prada's NYC headquarters I visit to get, as it were, a second opinion. 'Once you lose your hormones you are nothing more than roadkill. So you have two options. You can make a conscious decision that from now on, it is all about you, that you are going to do something you have never done before, which is put yourself first. Or you can continue in the way you want to continue until you drop dead. If you don't think that, explain to me why most older women who do not take hormones don't have their brains, are alcoholics, are fat and miserable, and impossible to live with. I've yet to see a woman in her sixties or seventies who's not on hormones who is doing something really wonderful unless she already had some major mission in life she wanted to achieve.'

The former director of a medical trauma

centre in upstate New York and a co-founder of the Bioidentical Hormone Initiative, a non-profit organisation dedicated to training doctors in how to treat age-related hormonal imbalances, Schwartz is also the founder of Evolved Science, a members-only preventive healthcare service (a branch has recently opened in London's Belgravia).

On the window sill in her New York office are pictures of children – I assume they are her children but in fact they are her grandchildren. Dressed in a tight black dress and Acne platform heels, Schwartz is a hybrid, kind of, of Joan Rivers and Charlize Theron and looks shockingly young for her age… which is 65.

I reiterate my concerns about having had oestrogen-positive breast cancer. 'Listen, lemme tell you something,' she says, crossing and uncrossing her shapely bare legs. 'If you *don't* take hormones you are going to wind up in trouble from every point of view. Brain. Bone. Heart. Your cancer. Not *your* cancer, because you never own cancer, but let me tell you, you didn't get breast cancer because you had too many hormones in your body. There are a million other reasons why you got cancer and one of them is that as you get older, your risk of cancer goes up independent of anything else. Even with Premarin, your risk of cancer goes down. Even with *them*, I'm saying you are better off [on the cancer front]. With oestrodil [that's the oestrogen derived from plant sources] you can *really* bring it down.

'Look,' she goes on, pausing briefly to point out the figure of Donald Trump emerging onto a balcony on the opposite building, 'nobody actually knows the significance of oestrogen-positive cancer. Scientifically, it is used as a bit of an intimidation tactic. Is it fuelled by oestrogen or is it that you need more oestrogen? What kind of oestrogen…?'

When I get back to London I have made my decision. Dr Schwartz has gone on record saying she thinks swine flu is nothing more than a common cold, but she has an immensely encouraging, not to say reassuring, vibe about her. Plus, she looks bloody marvellous for 65. I go to my local chemist to get my prescription. It costs me £40 for three months' worth.

There are three potions: Oestrogel (which mimics the oestradiol produced by the human ovary), Testim (another topical gel containing the androgen, testosterone) and Utrogestan (a capsule that contains the progesterone).

The first two have to be rubbed into my stomach and inner thighs once a day. The third, the progesterone, to 'oppose' the oestrogen, is to be taken the first seven days of every month (at night because it can cause drowsiness). For the first 24 hours I can't help feeling like Alice in Wonderland, wondering which potion is going to affect me in what way. Oestrogen and progesterone, fair enough, I was on the mini-pill before going off to university in the late 70s... for about a week. But testosterone? As my children's

So what was I going to do with this niggling 'tickle' the testosterone was giving me? The return of desire is all very well but every day, all day? As my friend Rosa put it, 'Do I actually need it 24/7? Frankly, I've not got the time.'

nanny wants to know, is it going to make me look like Fatima Whitbread? And, as I want to know, is it going to make me wanty to mounty the postman? What about the novel I thought I never had in me? What about acquiring a taste for theatre and poetry or perhaps even gardening? What about working on becoming, if not one of the leading thinkers of the 21st century, then at least the person my dog, if I had one, believed me to be? And for the next couple of days I cannot stop thinking about what this stuff is going to do to me – to the point, almost, of seeing things that are not there. The Ideal Hormones Show at Earls Court, and so on. And then, inevitably, I kind of forget, until about three weeks later, I realise the sleeplessness and hot flushes have disappeared. So, too, have the ridges on my nails (young nails, who knew of such a thing), although it doesn't do anything for my saggy earlobes (yes, sigh, earlobes sag with age).

Within a month I get my period back (oh, did I not tell you? Progesterone can give you a chemical bleed, the reason why it is entirely possible to 'menstruate' well into your seventies). Within three months (and, because I was feeling quite woozy with the progesterone, we had taken it down to seven days every alternate month, and we'd reduced the two pumps of Oestrogel to one), my meaty menopot, that extra duvet tog that seemingly had nothing to do with diet, had gone. If I overate, it came back, but it was *accounted* for, which made all the difference. I felt like my old self once again. Although, when I say 'old' self, what do I mean?

This even hormonal keel was *better* than my old self. Much better. On the other hand, what was I going to do with all the saucy dreams, and this niggling 'tickle' the testosterone was giving me? The return of desire is all very well. But every day, all day? As my friend Rosa put it, 'I suppose it's quite a fun thing to try, to put that particular libidinous hat on for two or three weeks, but do I actually need it 24/7? Frankly, I've not got the time.'

7

SEX, SILVER LININGS AND AMBITION

In talking about sex, it may be instructive to talk about the *peri*-menopause. The drink, as it were, in the last-chance saloon. The sun before it goes behind a very, very big cloud. Or, to put it more bluntly, those last remaining years when you can still have babies and your body is telling you to get out there and mate with someone, anyone, really, before it is too late.

It can be a grey area, that time leading up to the change. The average length is four years, but for some women it's a question of months, for others it may continue for ten years. Mine was somewhere in the middle and possible to identify properly only in retrospect. The one thing I did notice at the time was how my periods, after having been so erratic right from the get-go, suddenly got iron-clad regular, almost to the hour, but instead of being four weeks apart were now nearer three. Little did I know that this was my body giving me as many opportunities to reproduce as possible. It's hard not to look at that body now with a degree of affection, thinking how desperate it was to achieve this. During these last two years, the flow was so heavy that no ST in the world was going to stem it – I needed a small mattress. The cramps got really bad, too, a sign that my progesterone levels were dwindling.

Typically, it is in the last one to two years that the decline in oestrogen and progesterone accelerates, thereby giving temporary dominance to testosterone, the last of the hormonal troika to tail off. That's the 'male' androgen produced by our ovaries, adrenal glands and fat cells, which supposedly makes us pushier, hairier and, crucially, hornier… though not necessarily for the partner we've lived with and loved and watched growing man boobs for the past however many years.

'It happened like clockwork, to a group of us right before we hit 50,' explains 55-year-old music producer Sarah, 'we felt like a real demographic, so we called ourselves the 49ers. I'd got to a point where I knew no one was going to rip my clothes off in a fit of lust ever again and I just wasn't ready to say goodbye to that feeling. I suppose I'd gotten to the stage in my life where I didn't really care about the consequences and I went a bit mad, wearing glittery eye make-up, sleeping with much younger men, taking drugs and generally trying to keep the party going for as long as possible. Now I'm out of it, I can pick a 49er out in a crowd instantly. It's a real look: a hunter but at the same time slightly hunted.'

'Looking back it seems rather pathetic: older woman – too old to be a cougar, in fact – on the pull, but at the time, it was so exciting,' says another friend, a writer, now 55 and a year into menopause proper. 'It almost felt like I was making up for lost time, wanting to have those golden sexual experiences I never had at college or in my twenties because I was so screwed up about my body and too frightened and embarrassed to ask for what I wanted.

'I wasn't bogged down with childcare, I felt more confident about myself and my body than I'd ever done in my life, having managed to get down to the weight I was before I had kids. I couldn't remember the last time someone of the opposite sex had made a pass at me, so when it happened it was like a light being switched on. Or more like a flower blossoming in time-release photography. I'd always thought it quite crummy, the idea of cheating, and yet here I was doing just that. I couldn't bear the idea of going to my deathbed never having slept with anyone other than my husband ever again. To be really honest, I couldn't bear the idea of sleeping with my husband again.'

If oestrogen is the hormone of compliance, the 'Ladybird mum' hormone as one friend of mine describes it, then testosterone is the hormone of infidelity. It is also the hormone of novelty. Meaning, if you suddenly find yourself seeing the personal trainer in a whole new light or, gah, thinking inappropriate thoughts about your 18-year-old son's friends, don't worry, it's all perfectly normal; there are others out there just like you.

'We're programmed to seek out an alpha male with the best possible genes, not the prince who's charmingly slumped at our side,' says psycho-pharmacologist Dr Julie Holland, author of *Moody Bitches: The Truth about the Drugs You're Taking, the Sleep You're Missing, the Sex You're Not Having and What's Really Making You Crazy*. 'Older women are more likely to get aroused when in the company of younger, novel, pheromone-secreting men. We naturally pursue youthful specimens because there is less chance of genetic damage in younger DNA.'

Not that everyone becomes a member of the 49er club. Nor do they lose their libido the moment they stop bleeding for good. Look at the author Diana Athill who famously had a voracious sexual appetite right up until her mid-seventies. If, however, you are in the throes of feeling like a sex-mad teenager all over again, I'd say enjoy it while you can. Because chances are, when your periods stop for good, so will all trace of sexual desire. And that can be for some of us, far above and beyond the weight gain and the hot flushes and the sleepless nights, the harshest toke of all.

'I suddenly realised everything that had motivated me had been towards erotic possibility and attraction and all that shit,' says Sarah. 'I didn't know what I was *for* any more. You think you are an individual and have a free will, but what I discovered was that I had been run by hormones and I couldn't argue with that. It was, at first, devastating to adjust to.'

If oestrogen is the hormone of compliance – the 'Ladybird mum' hormone – as one friend of mine describes it, then testosterone is the hormone of infidelity.

'I still remember that cold, panicky feeling of, *what*? But I love sex!' says my friend Anna, 54 (interestingly, one of the few women I talked to who considered sex the cornerstone of her relationship). 'And I'm really *good* at it. It felt like I was closed for business, like the end of the world.

Had that been my lot?'

This is where testosterone supplementation comes in, still a controversial subject in the US, where it has not been approved by the FDA for female use. (Although at least 26 different testosterone products have been licensed for male use in the US, if doctors want to prescribe them for female patients, they have to do it 'off label'.)

Not that testosterone is the only hormone responsible for our sex drive. Oestrogen is too. Our thyroid glands, they play a big part in our libido too. Nor is testosterone solely connected with sex drive. Like oestrogen (to which testosterone can be converted in both the female and male body), it has an effect on memory and cognitive skills and is connected with a possible decrease of beta-amyloid and plaque build-up in the brain, with some studies suggesting it might help prevent against Alzheimer's.

Testosterone levels in women have also been linked to better bone density and, in female athletes, to lower body fat and higher muscle mass. (I know, I perked up when I first heard about that, too.)

There is evidence it may aid in the protection of our hearts. In 2010, research published in the *Journal of Clinical Endocrinology & Metabolism* showed that post-menopausal women with low levels of testosterone had an increased risk of cardiovascular disease. Another small study found that women with heart failure gained physical strength and the 'ability to function properly' when they started to take a testosterone supplement. There is also evidence from researchers at Wright State University in Ohio that it might help protect against breast cancer.

A paper in *Maturitas*, the official journal of the European Menopause and Andropause Society, said in September 2013 that, while conventional combined HRT raises the risk of breast cancer slightly, the addition of testosterone appears to cut that risk significantly.

Bingo wings and thinning hair, leaky bladders and painful intercourse through vaginal dryness... anecdotally, it can help with all that too. Sounds too good to be true? Hell, look at Jane Fonda. If that's her secret, there has to be something there.

The main reason, though, that doctors

prescribe it (or its precursor, the steroid hormone DHEA) for their menopausal patients is for a flagging or non-existent libido, and for many women it has had a transformational effect. But is it the magic pill?

I have a friend who conceived a couple of years ago via IVF, and subsequently underwent the menopause at the age of 45, for which she was prescribed HRT. She is, she says, on the highest dose of testosterone the doctor will allow her to take as she is fairly new to her marriage and was keen to get back into the swing of things as soon as possible after the birth. 'But it hasn't done a thing,' she says. 'No effect whatsoever, as if I'm just one of those rare unlucky women – like those rare unlucky women for whom the epidural doesn't work. And sex was a fundamental part of my life before, so I really don't know what to do. I'm hoping it's because I am so in love with my baby, but a big part of me thinks, that's it, that's the end.'

Meanwhile, if testosterone is 100 per cent safe, why won't the FDA approve it for female use? Dr Mary Gallenburg, senior gynaecologist at the

Mayo Clinic in the US, for one, warns that long-term studies on its safety in menopausal women with a history of breast or uterine cancer or those who have cardiovascular or liver disease are still lacking. Furthermore, excessive doses in women, have been linked to male-pattern hair loss, adult acne, a deepening of the voice and even clitoromegaly (an abnormally enlarged clitoris).

Put off? Well, luckily there are alternatives. According to US sexual-health expert and urologist Dr Jennifer Berman, we ignore the aphrodisiacal effects of omega fatty acids – those found in salmon, avocado and blueberries – at our peril. To supplement that, there are all sorts of sophisticated new sexual aids on the market, many of which are available through her sister, Dr Laura Berman. Heard, for example, of the Eros machine? A suction device that you fit over your bits 'to increase blood flow to the clitoris and surrounding vulval areas which therefore enhances sensitivity'?

And what about mindset? It would be mad not to take that into account. For isn't desire just as much a brain as a body thing? And isn't it true that it wanes and waxes in exact proportion to mood and situation? As a recent study published in the Endocrine Society's *Journal of Clinical Endocrinology & Metabolism* revealed, levels of testosterone and naturally occurring hormones may actually play quite a limited role in driving menopausal women's libido.

'While levels of testosterone and other reproductive hormones were linked to women's feelings of desire and frequency of masturbation, our large-scale study suggests psycho-social factors influence many aspects of sexual function,' says one of the study's authors, John F. Randolph, Jr, MD, of the University of Michigan Medical School in Ann Arbor. 'A woman's emotional well-being and the quality of her intimate relationship are tremendously important contributors to sexual health.'

'People have this idea that hormones cause behaviour, and that may be true,' says Dr Julie Holland, a former head of the emergency department at New York's Bellevue Hospital, 'but just as often environment and behaviour will actually trigger hormones. It may be that our husbands and partners aren't doing that for us. Say you start working out with a cute personal trainer, you're like, oh my God! I'm aroused! Well, his hormones are triggering your testosterone... which is why I tell my patients, even though you aren't feeling horny, go ahead and start having sex. Sometimes, even though you don't think you are in the mood, once you get going, things change.'

Or as the French poet Rabelais once said, '*L'appétit vient en mangeant...*'* I confess, though, that as I write this, I can feel a slight slump in the shoulders. This burden society puts on us older folk to bonk like 20-year-olds, is that the price we pay for living longer? My standard answer when a mere acquaintance wants to know about my sex life is: 'We've managed to limit it to once a day, thanks for asking,' which usually shuts them up.

But what gave them the right to ask in the first place? In a way, I wish it was like it was in the days of *The Lucille Ball Show*, i.e. when it was normal for couples with kids in their late teens to have separate beds; when it was okay for our sex lives,

* 'Appetite comes with eating...'

or the lack of them, to remain private. There has to be a reason, after all, why children retch at the idea of their parents having sex. So why do we find it so hard to admit not just to our friends but also to our doctors that that part of the relationship disappeared years ago?

'I was shocked when I went back to my doctor after being prescribed HRT and straight off, he asked me about my sex life, and wasn't it amazing how testosterone made orgasms so much deeper and quicker,' says Kate. 'And I had to tell him that my husband, whom I adored, and I hadn't had sex for years.

'When he then said why didn't I take a lover, like so very many of his other clients had, I was confused and a little offended. Should I – when I'd sort of put all that to bed, and was fine with it?'

This testimony struck a chord with me, on the testosterone. To have that level of desire when it is not necessarily directed at the person it is supposed to be directed towards didn't feel right. Somehow it just didn't seem fair, in my longstanding domestic situation, chemically destabilising the playing field, being in that permanent state of disconnect, and so, somewhat regretfully, after a month, I took myself off it.

When I hear stories from friends about the marvellous clandestine sex lives they are having, the stolen snogs in dark alleys, the filthy whatsapp conversations, the *cinq à sept* sessions in Premier Inns, yes, of course I feel a stab of something. Friends for whom sex has remained pivotal to the relationship, they stick in my craw, too. They stick in my craw because, yes, I do feel guilty at not having worked harder at the physical side of things, of so willingly taking the path of least resistance, of falling into the nice comfy trap of treating my partner like my sibling; of conflating intimacy, in a word, with familiarity. Perhaps, at this point, I should issue a clarion call to all you out there who still feel a teeny tiny iota of desire for your other halves. Keep that bathroom door closed! Have the dumb date nights! Role-play away! Because, like they say, once it has gone, it is almost impossible to get back.

On the other hand, it's kind of nice knowing that the hurly-burly of the chaise longue is history, that there is one thing less to think about as I go about my day. That I get out of bed in the morning and take pride in getting dressed not because my amygdala vainly hopes its carrier might still mate but just… because.

'I'd been menopausal for a year when I went to this very glamorous doctor in Cadogan Gardens who put me on HRT, including testosterone gel,' says Sarah. 'Within a week of being prescribed it, though, I had to come off it. It started reviving those feelings of sexual need which, after a year of not having them suddenly no longer felt appropriate. It felt inelegant, not mature. Within days I experienced this sort of bodily awareness, the edges of myself tingling, and I thought, do I like this? Is this right? And, in truth, being "unchained from the beast" was a weird kind of liberation. It's a small death, the menopause, and I'm still partially grieving, but if I don't feel authentic, I can't operate. And if my marriage of a quarter of a century cannot weather this, my way of thinking was, then what did that say? It was a *big* negotiation with my other half, but I had made a decision that I didn't want to live playing that game any more, that I *had* to go out and look for the silver-lining stuff. Yes, nature had been phenomenally cruel, but I had faith in nature and was sure there would be something else.'

My wise mother, who actively chose the single life after the breakdown of her last marriage and has flourished ever since, agrees. 'In these last 10 years I have felt quite unencumbered and free to do what I do,' she says. 'It's like giving up drinking or smoking – you don't have to think of taking your cigarettes or lighter with you, you don't have to worry about taking the car. Life becomes easier, simpler, not being in that game any more. But that is not to say you opt out completely. You are still in the game; it is just that it is a different game. I'm still competitive, maybe even more so, and let me tell you my main battles, if I have them, are more often than not with other women – the sisterhood is not the sisterhood when it comes to careers. But after years of it you do build up experience in dealing with these things – if you don't then you'd have to be pretty daft. There's also the notion that if it goes wrong, it doesn't matter and there's a kind of confidence in that…'

'There's a strange bullishness that takes over,' says Pippa, another 50-something friend. 'I always worried while in the thick of bringing up my children that I had peaked at 21 and it was downhill all the way, careerwise. I had become progressively less ambitious as my twenties, thirties and even forties passed. But now I can feel a little flame reigniting, almost in spite of myself. Having done years of mashed veg, and traipsing to the local swings, it's suddenly all about you, you as an island, self-sufficient in a way you haven't been for years – staying with your partner ideally because you love them, and enjoy them, but not because you need a hunter-gatherer to keep you in H & M children's clothes or to help heat the house any more.'

'That year when every scrap of oestrogen had left my body was definitely the year I discovered ambition,' says Sarah. 'That was when all that focus on being attractive and being in a sexual relationship shifted and I suddenly started fantasising about leadership and running companies. Which is not to say I lived like a housewife before, just that I'd never really been what you'd call pushy. And yet here I was thinking, fuck it, this is what is driving me now.'

8

MENOPAUSE AND MARRIAGE

'There is no more creative force in the world than a menopausal woman with zest.' So said the anthropologist Margaret Mead. 'PMZ', as a features writer recently dubbed it, although it could also be called PMD when you look at the latest divorce statistics.

I'd always thought it was the men who did the walking at midlife and beyond. That is what they do, don't they: trade us in for younger models, ideally going for someone with the same name so they don't have to repaint the boat's transom, and all?

Not necessarily. According to a landmark study conducted by *AARP* magazine, statistically it is us who are more likely to want out once the kids have left the nest, 66 per cent of us, in fact, leaving our poor menfolk walking around in a daze not knowing quite what hit them.* Post-divorce, it is also women who are more likely to appreciate their newfound freedom – men tend to report feeling better off after a divorce only when they have remarried. Not so much 'Dad, stop being so mean to Mum' then, as much as 'Mum, stop being so mean to Dad.'

Look, I'm not saying some men can't be shits. The long-suffering, selfless wife who gets dumped by her sub-standard husband after 20 years of marriage is hardly a niche demographic. But we can be pretty darn brutal too. And for every woman who descends into apologetic despair at this time of her life – maybe it's not the meno-pause, maybe it's just *me*?; for every woman who

---

* Study conducted in 2004, based on surveys with 1147 men and women between the ages of 40 and 79 who had gone through divorce in their forties, fifties and sixties. (http://assets.aarp.org/rgcenter/general/divorce.pdf)

doesn't think she's worth a bikini wax any more, who can't see the point in fixing the increasingly hillbilly teeth; for every woman who somehow believes because she has let herself go she doesn't deserve any better, there's another who feels that, actually, after years of dutifully putting supper on the table every single night and having sex with someone who now frankly repulses her, she damn well *does* deserve better. (The late-blooming lesbian: now that's another demographic, right there.)

The ancient Greeks had a whole philosophy about the menopause. When women reached 40, they were perceived to become drier, with the absence of blood, and (weirdly, given the hot flushes) colder. Because some women grew facial hair and their voices deepened around this age, the belief was that their physiology was becoming more male (and as we know, ancient Greeks always considered men's bodies to be far superior to women's anyway).

The question is, *do* we become more like men, once all the mummy hormones dribble away? Or do we become our true selves, the way God meant us to be, unchained from that wheel of reproduction and child-rearing?

It can certainly feel like that, for some of us. And according to American psychiatrist Louann Brizendine, MD, it has everything to do with our hormones. There's a biological equilibrium that we simply didn't have when we were menstruating, she explains in her book *The Female Brain*, what with our oestrogen and progesterone levels peaking and ebbing, depending on the time of the month – and if you took an MRI scan of a menopausal woman's brain you'd see the difference.

When those hormones are roller-coastering, she argues, the circuits between the amygdala (the bit of our brain associated with survival instincts, memory and emotions such as fear and sadness) and the pre-frontal cortex (the bit that regulates our behaviour and is most associated with abstract thought and making decisions) are constantly being over-amped. When those hormones dwindle, those circuits stop spiking and start running more consistently. That doesn't mean we become unfeeling automatons; it just means we can trust ourselves a bit more, knowing our realities aren't going to be drastically altered the way they so often were at certain times of the month. We don't think the end of the world is nigh just before we bleed.

Meanwhile, the decline in oestrogen causes our bodies to produce less oxytocin. And consequently, that urge to people-please the hell out of every situation, to avoid conflict at any cost, to 'want to help people and serve people and cut up their sandwiches into ever-tinier squares,' as the comedienne Sandra Loh Tsing put it in her cult menopausal memoir *The Mad Woman in The Volvo*, becomes radically less pronounced. It's as if nature is saying, if we can't have any more children, what is the point of instincts maternal or, for that matter, uxorial? What's the point of perpetually caving in and being so nice?

'You look at your husband and you think: it's my turn,' says a 55-year-old musician friend of mine, married with two grown-up children. 'For 25 years I've put your shirts in the washing machine, listened to you talking about your work and cooked you dinner. I worked out I've probably peeled and chopped 10,000 onions in the years we've spent together. That's an awful lot of onions.'

'I think way too little is said about the connection between hormones and nurturing,' she adds via email. 'The same hormones that keep you making spaghetti for your children's supper for two decades and driving bags full of tennis rackets back and forth – after the menopause, they switch off. This more or less coincides with your children heading off to university, which leaves just you and your husband

'I worked out I've probably peeled and chopped 10,000 onions in the years we've spent together. That's an awful lot of onions...'

alone in the house together. The last time you had this much time together, you were horny as anything and eager to soothe his troubled brow.

'But it's a different story now the oestrogen is wearing thin: the desire to look after him, to cook and take care of things, let alone do it – it just evaporates. No wonder you're ready for a gap year.

Or, more likely, a gap rest-of-your-life.'

So yes, we become, dare it be said, more like men.

Although, is that right? What about that woman who decides to take the 'gap-life'? As the *AARP* study revealed, 75 per cent of women who took the plunge enjoyed 'a serious, exclusive relationship after their divorce – often within two years.'

That's really heartening news, when one thinks of the husbands parading around their shiny new wives (or, indeed, yet another demographic here, their shiny new husbands), expecting their friends, their exes, their kids, to fall in as if nothing had happened. I know a few couples who fell madly in love with each other in their late fifties and sixties, and it is very encouraging, seeing them with this new lease of life, flirting with each other as if they were teens. Maybe menopause is precisely the time to bolt. Hell, maybe it should be compulsory.

But what about the woman who does just that and then realises she's made a terrible mistake? No study has been done on *that* particular demographic, not yet anyway, but surely there's a play, a short story – okay, a 1200-word feature – to be written about the woman who wakes up one morning in her two-up two-down in Shepherds Bush (as opposed to the rambling family home in Chelsea) next to the semi-professional karate instructor she left her husband and children for, who cannot believe the appalling error she has made?

'It was like a drug. I felt alive. Like a light had been switched on. And I couldn't see why it was wrong. I looked great, I felt great, I had this amazing tan, I felt I was really living and that I deserved it after 20 years of devoting myself to my kids and my husband. This was my time.' So speaks my friend Katy, California-based novelist and mother of three boys who, at the age of 49 – hah! Another 49-er! – found herself ready to end it all for a semi-professional tennis player she met while on assignment in Spain.

'What is scary, in retrospect, is how little empathy I had, how little guilt I felt; how, in the throes of peri-menopause, it seemed absolutely what I should I be doing. I remember thinking, this is really working, the kids seem really happy;

okay, my husband is a little miserable, but he's been happy for 20 years so he should just suck it up… I was, like, what else do you want? I'm here it's all good.

'I had no empathy for anyone, really. For example, there was this friend of mine who had just gotten brutally divorced after her husband met someone else at work. I got that she didn't like to be rejected, I got that the kids were upset, intellectually I understood the whole companionship thing, but emotionally I couldn't grab onto it. She was going to be single! She was going to find some cute guy with whom she could go to the movies and see the movies she wanted to see! She was going to be *free*.'

And then, she says, she got caught and she was forced to make a decision.

'A friend sent me to a therapist and I told her I might be on the verge of ruining my life, but I still didn't get it. I'd nod my head as she talked about intimacy and sharing and a deeper kind of love, and then the moment I walked out I'd be texting him. It really was like a fix, like I'd been chemically taken over. But eventually I quit him,

I still don't quite know how.'

Katy, now 53, is as immaculately turned out as ever in eau de nil cashmere and tracksuit bottoms, her earlobes and wrists discreetly glistening with diamonds. If you want to know what still-sexy-in-your-fifties looks like, Katy would be it. Four years on, after some serious rebuilding on her part, she is still with her husband and profoundly grateful for the way things turned out. Yes, she is now on hormones – a mixture of progesterone and DHEA (which promotes testosterone) – which she describes as 'helping things along... we still have sex – in fact we did it in the bathroom this morning. It's very different from "affair" sex – sometimes you come, sometimes you don't – but it always feels good.'

Regrets, though, does she have a few? 'I think it infuriates my husband I'm not more remorseful,' she says with a wry smile, 'but I can't erase it, I can't pretend it didn't happen. There will always be a part of me that rebels against the fact of monogamy and the notion that marriage ends a certain kind of ownership of our bodies and adventures.'

Katy is deeply grateful to the friend who recommended the therapist and knows for sure that it would have been a terrible idea to run off into the sunset with her lover 'who was, in retrospect, a pretty second-rate person.

'I look at it now as a choice between having almost everything – a wonderful, secure home and family, happy children, companionship and shared values and the joy of sharing books, music, friendships, extended family and history – but saying goodbye to the intoxication of selfish, self-reflective fantasy sex and the bubble of pure freedom.

'For some reason when I was in it that choice seemed possible and if I had acted on it my life would have been a very diminished, very self-oriented and ultimately, I think, very sad life... but that doesn't mean that I don't miss the moments of bliss. In the clutches of hormonal shifts and changes, the world looks a very different place and love and empathy get really wiped out – it is incredibly easy to make terrible mistakes.'

9

SOME THINKING ABOUT DRINKING

For many women, around the time they hit menopause, their tolerance for alcohol decreases. You hear it all the time. My one pleasure left in the world, a friend will moan, and I can't even enjoy that any more! Well, lucky them. Because my tolerance seemed to go up. And with HRT, unlike for a lot of women I know, it didn't abate. Where two glasses of wine used to be perfectly sufficient for an evening, now it was more like half a bottle, and quite often more.

But had my body built up a tolerance? Or had

rules simply got laxer, the 8pm threshold turning to 7pm and so on? The fact was that, by the time I hit my fifth decade, the hangovers were actually getting worse. They definitely exacerbated the hot flushes – it was almost psychosomatic; I could feel my body temperature rising with that first sip, especially with red wine – and my REM sleep, frankly, was fragmented as hell.

In retrospect, I think what I was doing was ploughing through. Alcohol was my link, sort of, to the hurly-burly of my thirties and forties, a reminder that I could still be, as it were, fun and gay; it gave a sense of occasion to an otherwise humdrum day. And being a feast or famine sort of person, the idea of cutting down to one small glass a day seemed almost more depressing than actually giving up. So I continued apace, desperately trying to recreate the effect drink used to have on me when I drank moderately, feeling more and more bloated and oyster-eyed and menopausal than ever.

This almost allergic reaction is not simply psychosomatic. From as young as 30 our bodies start changing composition. Generally what happens, whether we are male or female, is that we lose muscle mass and our fat content increases. Our body water levels drop, too, which not only makes for drier skin and wrinkles, but also means a lot of us, by the time we hit 50, are walking around dehydrated. When we drink alcohol, we become as sere as deserts inside. As we age, our livers get bigger but less efficient and the enzymes in our stomachs that help metabolise alcohol dwindle too, meaning alcohol hangs around in the body for longer, allowing more pure ethanol to go directly to our organs including the brain. (Alcohol has also been proved to exacerbate the natural cognitive decline we experience in our fifties and sixties when our neurons lose speed.)

Another thing to remember: alcohol is not stored in fat. When there is more fat in the body and less muscle mass, the alcohol is forced into the bloodstream, wreaking more damage. This is the reason why, generally speaking, women who have a higher fat to muscle ratio tend to handle alcohol less well than men.

For most menopausal women, then, alcohol seems to be a lose-lose situation, ironic when this is precisely the time when drink, in the face of all those other things we lose, can be such a comfort.

Red wine, with all its sulphites and tannins, can be particularly bothersome, which is why you see a lot of women my age hitting the tequila, the supposedly 'organic' spirit which doesn't give you a hangover.

My own mitigation involved drinking a lot more water (two litres a day minimum, because you can do crack cocaine as long as you hydrate adequately, as a New York fashion editor once told me in the 80s) and experimenting a bit on the wine front. For a while I decided to drink only biodynamic. A brand called Skinny Champagne – I was hooked on that for a time, too, until the ludicrous expense of it hit home. There was a phase of drinking anything I wanted as long as it was 11.5 per cent or under (and what a joyless, pointless phase that was). Then there was my long love affair with rosé. Preferably pale French rosé the colour of straw, chilled within an inch of its life, and enjoyed all year round, partly because it seemed more festive and sporty and outdoorsy than white and less heavy than red, but mostly because it slipped down so easily. (Rosé, it turns out, has a higher sugar content than either white or red and is the reason why so many of us come home from a lovely Mediterranean holiday feeling shit. Whispering Angel. Hah. Whispering Satan, more like, the amount I could put back.)

While all this strenuous mitigating was going on, I'd be on the constant look-out for studies linking moderate alcohol consumption to a reduced risk of cardiovascular problems, better bone density, etc. There's always one around somewhere if you look hard enough, just like there's always a report of sunshine somewhere, if you look hard enough, like on page 10 of Google, when every other weather channel is showing thunder and lightning.

Well? If oestrogen is supposed to have beneficial effects on your heart and bones, and if alcohol consumption is supposed to increase the oestrogen in your blood, then this moderate drinking would make wonderful sense.

Except the word 'moderate', the one that means one measly glass a day... In my case, there was no getting round that. Nor the evidence of alcohol's increasing, almost incontrovertible link with breast cancer. There was one study published by the *Journal of Women's Health* in 2012, suggesting that, in fact, red wine might help actually reduce breast cancer. Everyone jumped on that one, but it turned out to be teeny tiny – involving only 36 pre-menopausal women and lasting only a month.

My own mitigation involved drinking a lot more water, two litres a day minimum (because you can do crack cocaine as long as you hydrate adequately, as a New York fashion editor once told me)...

Another study carried out by Brigham and Women's Hospital in Boston, Massachusetts, in which the drinking habits of around 105,986 women were analysed between 1980 and 2008 came to the conclusion that around three to six glasses of wine a week raised a woman's risk of breast cancer by 15 per cent. (However, as critics pointed out when the study was published in 2011 in the *Journal of the American Medical Association*, if an average 50-year-old woman had a five-year breast cancer risk of around 3 per cent, a 15 per cent increase would raise that risk only to 3.45 per cent).

In a report published alongside the Brigham study, Dr Steven Narod of the Women's College Research Institute in Toronto concluded that women who consumed one drink a day would see their 10-year risk of breast cancer rise from 2.8 per cent to 3.5 per cent.* For women who had two drinks a day it would rise from 2.8 per cent to 4.1 per cent. That meant women who had, um, four drinks a day (and that is less than half a bottle) could be looking at 8.2 per cent. It made me think anew about the grape-seed-sized tumour I had found in my right breast that summer of 2007. Could it have been caused by my drinking? And now that I was on HRT, could I be putting myself in danger of getting it again? (The smart thing to do, according to Dr Martin Galy, a fashionable hormone doctor I went to see in London,

* Study started in 1976 and involved 105,000 women aged between 30 and 55

would be to reduce the drink and carry on with the HRT. He told me that, although he recommends only using bio-identical hormones, you are probably safer, both for protection of well-being and against cancer, taking even the most generic, sledge-hammering form of HRT than *not* taking HRT and continuing to drink in quantities greater than the recommended amount. And if that's not enough, the most recent NICE guidelines also reflect this advice.).

Although it was somewhat heartening to learn that once you've got your breast cancer, alcohol did not help the tumour to grow, it was really really hard to find a study that did not, in some way, link alcohol to getting breast cancer in the first place.

Which didn't curb my habit. At all. See, the more I drank, the more I *could* drink. To grossly misquote Aristotle: We are what we repeatedly do. Drinking, then, is not an act, but a habit.

An alcoholic? *Moi*? Well, something wasn't right. Something wasn't right if the idea of going out and not having a drink had become so appalling that I'd end up not going out. And then, er, opening a bottle anyway.

I suddenly realised the kids rarely saw me past 7.30pm without a glass of wine in my hand. I also realised how there would never be a situation, unless I was in bed with a fever, where I drank less than my other half. What had happened to that basic rule of thumb? That a woman in her twenties slurring her words and swaying a bit can be quite sweet? That a woman in her thirties can just about get away with it too? That a woman in her forties needs to watch out and that in her fifties it becomes, frankly, grotesque? How come I saw it in others, but not myself?

And then there came a point, in January 2016, to be precise, when I just stopped. I realised I'd done enough drinking in my life thanks very much, and I didn't want any more. I didn't want to be in that permanent low-level state of hung-overness, I didn't want my partner to feel that he had to constantly monitor me from the other end of the table, I didn't want to be obsessed with how slowly everybody drank compared to me, I didn't want to be more interested in the wine list than the menu. What I did want was to wake up feeling the same way I had done the night before, a feeling I hadn't experienced for what seemed an awfully long time, and the only way to do that was… to give it up.

You may not need to, and I envy you. The idea of a summer in Mykonos without rosé, of going to my favourite Italian restaurant without drinking red wine, of getting through a family Christmas without any medication at all is pretty unspeakable. Drinking *is* good for you in moderation. The experts (on page 10 of Google) *say* it is. But at the same time, if I'm going to make anything of this third third of my life, I'm probably going to have to do it sober. Wish me luck.

10

A LITTLE BIT OF NEW SCIENCE

In terms of medical innovation, I'm afraid we're not that sexy or urgent a demographic. We ought to be – by 2020 there will be 60 million peri- and post-menopausal women living in the US alone – but we are not. Not yet anyway. Companies like Calico, Human Longevity Inc et al are obsessed with making death optional, ploughing billions into cures for cancer, diabetes and heart disease, but when it comes to hot flushes and meno-pots and dry vaginas, meh, we need to get over ourselves. Or so it feels.

There is part of me that feels that, actually, we

probably do need to get over ourselves. Why medicalise something that is so perfectly natural? Why not ride it out, as so many of our mothers did, and be emotionally stronger for it on the other side? Isn't this just another First World problem? Do the Hadza women of Tanzania complain about hot flushes? And besides, how are we going to change the way the world views older women if, at 55, we expect to look and feel as though we were 40?

On the other hand, if average life expectancy for a woman is 85 and going up all the time, if – assuming the age we become menopausal pretty much stays put – we can expect to live more than a third of our lives in a post-reproductive state, is it intelligent or right that we should live it with crumbling bones and poor memory and a general 'it'll do' approach to the way we look and feel? Biologically, wouldn't that not add up?

It's hard not to feel that if men got the menopause like we got the menopause, a cure for hot flushes and irritability without the risk of cancer would have been invented ages ago. Gloria Steinem was so right when she said back in the

60s that if guys could get pregnant 'abortion would be a sacrament'.

It's not all bad. Take a treatment, currently in development, that could administer oestrogen to our brains only, therefore bypassing the potentially dangerous side effects on our uteri and breasts and so forth. The chemical, discovered by Professor Laszlo Prokai, the Robert A. Welch Chair in Biochemistry at the University of North Texas Health Science Center, is called DHED (an acronym given from the chemical name of the molecule) and is nearly identical to natural human oestrogen, except that it has an extra oxygen atom. Prokai's study found that a specialised protein found in rats' brains recognises the chemical and chops off the oxygen, turning DHED into oestrogen – whereas the body's other organs lack this protein so they can't turn DHED into oestrogen. When rodents, bred for use as experimental animals with their ovaries removed to mimic menopause, were administered this 'prodrug', there was a measurable increase of oestrogen in the brain but *not* in the uterus or bloodstream. Furthermore, as Prokai and his colleagues found, unlike oestrogen, DHED did not appear to promote the growth of breast cancer cells in culture or when implanted into mice. The potential upshot? The disappearance of hot flushes and symptoms of depression or cognitive impairment *without* an increased risk of cancer. DHED has not been tested on humans and thus requires development costing over a billion dollars and lasting several years to gain approval as new medication.

In fact, though it may not seem like it, tremendous leaps and bounds have been made on our behalf in the last 10 to 15 years; it's just that they weren't necessarily made in the name of boring old menopause; they were made in the much more exciting and urgent name of reproduction and (in)fertility.

Controversial biomedical gerontologist and Cambridge professor, Aubrey de Grey, for one, has already stated that the menopause could be 'cured' by stem cell science and regenerative therapy within 20 years. 'We could rejuvenate the ovary by stimulating or replenishing stem cells,' de Grey told the *Times* in 2014. 'We could create a whole new ovary through tissue-engineering like an artificial heart. There are all manner of possibilities.'

Sounds a bit Brave New World-y? All medical breakthroughs do at first. And de Grey (who, let's remember, has also claimed that the first 1000-year-old has already been born) is not the only one predicting a world where we'll be able to conceive well into our late fifties and beyond. Take Jonathan Tilly, a reproductive biologist from Harvard Medical School who came up with a remarkable discovery in 2004.

'We want women to study, have careers, be in boardrooms like men, but women still have to do all this during what is the most fertile period of their life. So if we are going to live longer, healthier lives after what is now our natural reproductive life, we are going to need changes.'

In the process of analysing the lifespan of cells, he isolated a population of rare 'oogonial stem cells' in rodents' ovaries, which were capable of producing a constant supply of fresh eggs or oocytes – therefore totally upending the widely held dogma that women are born with a finite number of eggs and that by the time we reach the menopause they have all disappeared. (The time when we have the most, around seven million, is when we are five-month-old foetuses in our mothers' bellies, from which point, tragically, it all goes downhill.)

That paper of Tilly's was heavily criticised by the medical science community when it came out, but it was supported by a study performed in China in 2009. Biologists led by Ji Wu at Shanghai Jiao Tong University claimed they had isolated a population of stem cells in adult female mouse ovaries, which they used to produce mature egg cells. These eggs, which had been injected with fluorescent green protein to identify them, successfully fertilised and resulted, yes, in glowing green offspring...

It was music to Tilly's ears, though it took him a few years to take the research one step further. Thanks to his colleague, Yasushi Takai of Saitama Medical University in Japan, he was able, this time, to prove to the doubting Thomases that those precious 'oogonial' stem cells existed in humans as well as rats. How? Because Takai had in his lab, at Tilly's disposal, ovary tissue donated by six healthy young Japanese women in the process of undergoing gender reassignment surgery. Using Ji Wu's protocol, Tilly and his team managed to extract those oogonial stem cells from the donated tissue, and after treating them with the green fluorescent protein, implanted them in the sterilised mice. Between 10 and 14 days later, they saw that immature follicles had formed... with glowing green oocytes in the middle of them. As Tilly said at the time, 'It made the hairs on my arm stand up.'

Tilly now holds a patent on human egg stem cells, and with the help of reproductive biologist Evelyn Telfer from the University of Edinburgh (who has pioneered a procedure to bring those egg cells to full maturity, which is exactly where Tilly's work has come to a halt), he hopes to radically change the current approach to fertility treatment as well as to incurable diseases such as Parkinson's.

He has also potentially rewritten the rules about how we women age. If Tilly's trajectory continues in the way he hopes, our ovaries could eventually keep working until the end of our lives.

Ethical and legal implications aside, imagine what that would be like: to be able to delay or even reverse the menopause; to bypass hot flushes and night sweats and osteoporosis; to remain as healthy and glossy-haired and pliable-boned as we were in our twenties and thirties... and that's without the sword of cancer hanging over our heads.

Imagine, for God's sake, being able to sprog again? Because that's the logical trajectory, isn't it? Forget about the Sandwich Years, as they are called. This will be the age of the Triple Decker, what with the parents who won't die, the school leavers who won't leave *and* a new baby or two.

'Of course, we are more likely to think that what is the norm is natural, because that is what has always happened, but if we are looking at a future where women are going to be living to 100, where for half our lives our ovaries don't work, then people are going to want a new normal. So there are going to have to be social changes, but technology will also have an increasingly important place.'

So speaks geneticist and molecular biologist Aarathi Prasad, 40, the glamorous author of *Like A Virgin: How Science Is Redefining the Rules of Sex*, and presenter of the recent Radio 4 feature, 'Rewinding the Menopause'. In the programme, which aired in 2015, she looked into how all this new research into fertility can help stave off the menopause and how society is going to deal with that.

Should we be greedily availing ourselves of all this new technology, aimed, let's face it, at young women in premature menopause, desperate to conceive? Or should we be going gently into this particular good night and gracefully accepting our lot? Just like our mothers did. And their mothers did. And their mothers before them. And look at them. They just about managed, didn't they?

Interestingly, a lot of the menopausal women Prasad approached for the interview either refused to participate, or insisted on remaining anonymous. God forbid it should seem like we're complaining, sort of thing. Older women complaining. So boring, after all. Although sometimes I wonder if we are our own worst enemies, the way we can gang up on each other for not being tougher, the way we can pull a 'Gaslight' on ourselves, colluding with the old patriarchal mindset that most women are mad anyway...

Prasad raised a few hackles at the Hay Festival in 2015 when she quoted scientists who say that the menopause has become 'abnormal' – that in the modern world, where resources are plentiful and we are living longer, healthier lives (and older women don't need to stop breeding in order to forage for food), it is redundant to our needs and it may be that evolution does away with it.

'Some scientists say that humans have already evolved as far as we are going to,' she says over coffee near her office at University College London, 'because, rather than us adapting to our environment, what we have become good at is adapting our environments to us. Evolution may or may not be a trajectory which has finished, but to live a third of your life when the rest of your body is functioning perfectly but your ovaries are not is referred to by some doctors as living with organ failure, and the consequences of this clock don't fit with the way we live in the modern world.

'We want women to study, have careers, be in boardrooms like men, but women still have to do all this during what is the most fertile period of their life. So if we are going to live longer, healthier lives after what is now our natural reproductive life, we are going to need changes. Forty-five may not be considered too old to have a baby nowadays, but medicine still refers to women as older mothers after the age of 35. That's because our eggs accumulate mutations as we age, which tends to mean they will be less healthy, so we become increasingly less likely to conceive or bring a baby to term the closer we get to the menopause.

'A woman came up to me at the end of my talk at Hay saying she loved being menopausal, being free of having periods or getting pregnant. At another talk, an older woman asked why people might not want to go through something so natural as the menopause. But there are plenty of things we do today that avert the natural: pacemakers, or keeping premature babies in incubators. We have seen that, when new reproductive technologies are available, people do seek them out. That is something that is only likely to increase in future. Education, getting a suitable job, being able to afford a house, schooling, all these things are happening later in life now. People are putting off having families for good reasons. And technological solutions will have to be sought if, more and more, we are going to want to have our families later in life.'

It's funny. One of the ironic upshots of the menopause is that I have suddenly become weirdly broody – broody in a way I never was before, during or after having kids.

It's no secret to anyone who knows me that I've always preferred dogs to children. Since I hit the menopause, though, I've begun looking at babies in the street in an entirely different way (and *here* is a little dirty secret, suddenly regretting I never even bothered to breastfeed the second one). In a way it makes a certain societal sense. I'm as established as I'm ever going to be in my career. I have a totally stable partner. I've got tons more patience. And even if I didn't, I've got the help to pick up the slack. Wouldn't it make sense to become a mother now, as opposed to then, when I had so much else on my plate?

And then I play it forward a little. It's one thing, a 70-year-old dad at the school gates in his Prada sneakers and his baseball cap. But a 70-year-old mum? That is something altogether different. Then again, why should 60 be an unnatural age to have a baby if we are going to live until we are 120? And, like Prasad says, who says natural is best anyway? The mother whose baby would have died if she hadn't had a caesarean? The cancer patient undergoing radio- or chemotherapy? The couple who have just been told that the 10th bout of IVF has worked?

Look, the idea of a mother and daughter-in-law two-fer-one special at the Portland doesn't appeal in the least, but the idea of feeling the way I do now on the hormones, for the next quarter of a century or more, with no fear whatsoever of my cancer returning? Oh, yes please. I'd take that like a shot.

ACCEPTANCE, ANDY WARHOL
AND A POEM

As I write this I am thinking about something my 13-year-old son told me over the weekend. 'Mum?' he went. 'Do you realise you've got really long hairs growing out of your nose?' The awful thing is, the little s*** is right. It appears I do.

And like the rogue eyebrow hairs which, however much you pluck them, always corkscrew back, stronger, whiter and more professorial than ever, they haven't always been there. It's not so much that I'm morphing into my mother, I'm morphing into her *father*, (my grandfather), it sometimes feels. Then there's my male-pattern baldness. Okay, an exaggeration, but when I look at pictures of my hair from a few years ago, I'm shocked by how thick and bouncy it was compared to what it is now. Those elastic pony-tail holders? Once upon a time I could only get them round twice. Now they'll easily go round three times. The scary thing is, if I bite the bullet, surrender to the truth and get myself one of those short grown-up haircuts, I'll probably never ever grow it long again. No more speed-plaiting strands of it when I'm bored or anxious, then; no more being able to put it up with a pencil and then taking out it for effect. Which, if I'm brutally honest with myself, may be no bad thing, no bad thing at all. There are very, very few women in their fifties who can get away with nearly waist-length hair. Moores, Julianne and Demi. That's about it.

Writing a conclusion is tricky. What are the take-home messages etc, etc... Someone asked me recently, if I had my druthers, would I have 'done' menopause differently? Well, maybe I would have stuck my head in the sand less and prepped more. Given up drink earlier. Bought the bigger-sized jeans. Gotten the grown-up haircut.

Approached it like my friend and yoga teacher Nadia who, at 43, doesn't feel nearly there yet, but who is determined not to get 'caught short' when it happens. I admire her prophylactic strategy. And her steadfast refusal to see menopause in a negative light.

A lot of the work, Nadia believes, is about learning to accept herself now, as she is, no matter what. (As yet she is childless and without a long-term partner). 'I need to be okay with the way things are as they are and continue to be okay, however it pans out to be for me,' she says. 'Who knows what will happen in the next five, ten years, but I don't want to enter the last third of my life with any trace of bitterness or regret. There are two ways to age, one is to be brittle and unyielding, the other is to be fluid and flexible, I'd like to be the latter...'

The kids or marriage thing? She's not ruling that out (or in) either. 'Plenty of middle-aged mothers I know are dissatisfied,' she shrugs, 'The point is, you've got to find joy and contentment with whatever life brings you.

'I have a friend who is 49 and in a reasonably

new relationship,' she goes on. 'Her partner offered to go down the IVF route, before it was really too late, because he knew she wanted a child. But when she sat down and really thought about it, after years of feeling resentful that she might never be a mother, she realised she was fine as she was. There's a kind of elegance with that kind of acceptance, I think.'

Nadia is very beautiful, with a killer, *killer* body – imagine a brunette Bo Derek – so I'm curious how she'll deal on the looks front. (Her mother, who was also very beautiful, had a face-lift at 40). 'Look, you can be sexy without that being your main currency. Once upon a time, yes, I did turn heads when I walked into a room; I don't do that any more, but that's okay. You have to relinquish that kind of power and replace it with something else. I'm sure that's why so many women turn to yoga in middle age, filling themselves from the inside rather than the other way round. You *can't* go into that next stage filled with regret and thinking, what did I do wrong? You have to enter it with a degree of grace.'

Grace. If there is one word that seems important

at this stage of my life it is this one. And when I think of the women (and men) I talked to while researching this little book, *that's* the quality which always shines out. Shit happens. You deal. With as much humour and style and acceptance as you can muster.

About seven years ago I had my passport stolen in Boston airport and had to get a new one in a hurry in order to be let back into the UK. I got the photo done in some booth in a mall on Cape Cod. My mother and I had had a row about something or other just before it was taken. And I remember thinking at the time, that has to be the worst picture that has ever been taken of me: how could I look so weathered and old and cross? I've had to renew my passport since, but keep the old clipped one in my top drawer. Passport photos are such life markers somehow. The other day I had a look inside and was shocked with... well, how marvellous I looked. Am I going to think that, ten years from now, of my current passport picture? I showed it to a friend of mine recently. 'Who is that man?' she said.

There is a part of me which rather resents

younger women, women in their thirties and early forties, who've reached the sweet spot of their lives and (like me at that age) couldn't be less interested in the subject of menopause. I want to shake my fist and tell them, 'It'll come to you soon enough!' But then there is another part of me that is excited for them, excited for *myself*, for what is to come. Whether it is a function of menopause or not, I trust myself more, I like myself more, I'm not quite as fearful of what life might or might not toss out. So what if I inadvertently offend someone? So what if I don't get invited to the party?

'Sometimes people let the same problem make them miserable for years when they could just say, "So what". That's one of my favourite things to say. "So what",' as Andy Warhol once said.

Look. There's a fine balance between being liberated and giving up – and I'm still learning how to walk it (still learning to accept that word 'balance' actually); but, if there is any time in my life when the penny drops and I'm going to get it, now is that time.

What the hell are we here for, what's the point

of us; once we die, is that it? The older you get the louder these questions become. Sometimes to stop them deafening me I like to remember the etymological definition of the word 'ecstasy'. It comes from the ancient Greek and means, literally, to stand outside of the self ('ek' meaning outside of, and 'stasis' – stature, standing). There we are. True bliss is to get over ourselves. To quote Bertrand Russell from *The Conquest of Happiness*, one of the greatest self-help books of all time: 'One of the symptoms of an approaching nervous breakdown is the belief that one's work is terribly important.'

One's work. One's self. One's reflection in the mirror while trying on bikinis. It all sort of boils down to the same thing. There's a life out there beyond *me*, and I'm game to explore it.

Is this a good conclusion? Maybe that's the point: it isn't a conclusion. Whatever the case, here is something from the Sufi poet Rumi, about s*** happening and accepting it with grace, which feels an appropriate way to sign off:

The Guest House
by Mewlana Jalaluddin Rumi

This being human is a guest house.
Every morning a new arrival.

A joy, a depression, a meanness,
some momentary awareness comes
As an unexpected visitor.

Welcome and entertain them all!
Even if they're a crowd of sorrows,
who violently sweep your house
empty of its furniture,
still treat each guest honorably.
He may be clearing you out
for some new delight.

The dark thought, the shame, the malice,
meet them at the door laughing,
and invite them in.

Be grateful for whoever comes,
because each has been sent
as a guide from beyond.

AUTHOR BIOGRAPHY

D'Souza has written for publications such as the *Guardian*, the *Daily Mail*, the *Times*, the *Daily Telegraph*, *Vanity Fair*, and the *Evening Standard*, and is currently contributing editor of British *Vogue*. In her articles, she often probes body issues such as ageing, weight-control, diet, cosmetic surgery, and her own battle with cancer. She lives in London, with her partner and two sons.